The Early
Development of
Xenopus Laevis

Peter Hausen
Metta Riebesell

The Early Development of Xenopus Laevis

An Atlas of the Histology

With 64 Figures and 43 Plates

Verlag der Zeitschrift
für Naturforschung
Tübingen

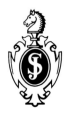

Springer-Verlag
Berlin Heidelberg New York
London Paris Tokyo Hong Kong
Barcelona Budapest

Professor Dr. Peter Hausen
Max-Planck-Institut für Entwicklungsbiologie
Abteilung V für Zellbiologie
Spemannstraße 35/V, 7400 Tübingen, FRG

Metta Riebesell
Max-Planck-Institut für Entwicklungsbiologie
Abteilung V für Zellbiologie
Spemannstraße 35/V, 7400 Tübingen, FRG

Distributed by Springer-Verlag Berlin Heidelberg New York

ISBN 3-540-53740-6 Springer-Verlag Berlin Heidelberg New York
ISBN 0-387-53740-6 Springer-Verlag New York Berlin Heidelberg

Library of Congress Cataloging-in-Publication Data. Hausen, Peter, 1935–. The early development of Xenopus laevis : an atlas of the histology / Peter Hausen, Metta Riebesell. p. cm. ISBN 3-540-53740-6. – ISBN 0-387-53740-6. 1. Xenopus laevis–Development–Atlases. 2. Xenopus laevis–Histology–Atlases. I. Riebesell, Metta, 1954–. II. Title. QL668.E265H38. 1991. 597.8′4–dc20 91-13585

Typesetting, printing and binding: Allgäuer Zeitungsverlag GmbH, Kempten
31/3145-543210 – Printed on acid-free paper

Preface

When development commences in the fertilized egg countless processes are integrated and canalized to generate the well ordered increase in complexity which culminates in the emergence of the macroscopic spatial pattern of the embryo. Research in embryology is pursued on all organizational levels of the system with the common aim being to answer the question as to how this macroscopic pattern is generated. Since cells are the building elements of the structures generated, the question may be rephrased: How do cells cooperate to produce supracellular structures and further, what are the controlling mechanisms which make them behave this way? Most of the studies performed in developmental biology are ultimately related to these questions and, in fact, have their origin in observations at the cellular level.

For this reason morphological studies at the cellular level of a developmental process are required before one can embark on the analysis of the subcellular or molecular processes involved. This top-down strategy helps to define the relevant questions and provides guidelines for further detailed studies. This book is intended as an aid to this strategy.

The collection of photographs presented here aims to provide a comprehensive overview of the morphogenesis of the early *Xenopus* embryo. The reproductions give an insight into the multitude of the intracellular events during oogenesis and illustrate the sophisticated behavior of the cells as they later cooperate to gradually form the basic body plan of the embryo.

Most of the relevant morphological features have been amply described in the vast literature on amphibian development over the past 100 years, but their pictorial presentations are widely scattered and the individual communications are mostly concerned with special details which encompass only a small section of the entire process. The present collection of plates may help the reader to follow, in the context of the whole, the individual traits through prolonged periods of their development.

Furthermore, the new histological techniques applied here yield sections of a quality and resolution which are rarely met in the older literature. Our own need for detailed histological information resulted from current laboratory work. Results from immunostainings or in situ hybridizations are notoriously difficult to interpret due to the poor preservation of the histological sections used in these methods. A precise knowledge of the histological structure of the embryo at different stages of development was found to be of great help. These experiences and considerations encouraged us to undertake the effort of publishing this atlas of the histology of early *Xenopus* development.

The interpretation of the plates requires a basic knowledge of the processes that occur during development. The accompanying text is intended to provide an aid for the proper appreciation of the plates.

In this text embryogenesis is viewed as an epigenetic process in the traditional sense of the term: a continuous succession of structural transformations in which each newly emerging feature has its origin in the topographical and functional organization of the preceding phase, and every change in organization provides the basis for the further elaboration of the structural wealth of the organism. A satisfying view of such a system is obtained only when at each stage the history of a structure is given the same attention as its future fate. In fact, many processes or structures become understandable only in this framework of temporal relations. For these reasons it is difficult to describe the development of an organism by simply following the time axis. It seems inevitable to move back and forth in time to view and analyze the emergence and elaboration of the individual traits of the system and to try to integrate these into the network of the whole. The text is arranged much in this way.

This essay is not intended as a comprehensive review. Such reviews which cover the field of amphibian embryogenesis exhaustively have recently been published. Neither is it meant to be a critical review. In this field many of the explanations proposed are, in fact, much disputed and many experimental observations are open to differing interpretations. To follow all these arguments would have unduly lengthened this work making it too difficult to read. Instead, we have chosen to provide a general view and have attempted to present the consensus opinion on the most prominent features and traits. The text gives an introduction to the field and together with the plates provides a kind of traveler's guide through the landscape of *Xenopus* embryogenesis. Wherever possible, the reader is referred to the photographic plates, and terms which are used in the explanatory drawings are printed in bold face in the text when they are mentioned for the first time. References are not cited in the text, but reviews are given at the end of each chapter together with references of some original articles which are dealt with in the text but are not explicitly treated in the reviews cited. The collection of references should allow easy access to the literature for more detailed inquiries.

In the interest of brevity, the whole field of molecular biology of *Xenopus* development has been, with a few exceptions necessary for a basic understanding, largely neglected. A description of the fast growing and changing area of molecular research would require many additional considerations, and the pathway bridging the gap between the molecular field and the main topic of this text, which is the development of *Xenopus* as it is seen at the cellular level, leads too often through unsafe and sometimes impassable terrain.

Acknowledgments

We are particularly grateful to Peter D. Nieuwkoop for carefully reading the manuscript and for many comments. His help in interpreting the plates was invaluable. Rudolf Winklbauer has critically read the manuscript and has accompanied the emergence of the work with continuous interest and helpful suggestions. We wish to express our gratitude. We also acknowledge the cooperation of Daniel St. Johnston, who has guided us through the pitfalls of English grammar and semantics. Ursula Müller worked out the initial details of the histological procedures, Doris Eder carefully helped on the graphical part, Wolf Kergl carried out the explanatory drawings of the gastrulation, and Roswitha Grömke-Lutz worked on the phototechnical part. They all deserve our gratitude. Our particular thanks are also dedicated to Margot Heller for typing the manuscript. We are indebted to the many coworkers in the Max-Planck-Institut für Entwicklungsbiologie for fruitful and critical discussions without which this work could not have been completed.

Tübingen, March 1990   *P. Hausen*
                                         M. Riebesell

Contents

An Outline
of Xenopus Development

Chapter 1
Introduction

As a precondition for any analytical work on the development of an embryo, a framework of orientation has to be established by dividing the continuous developmental process into a succession of phases, each defined by some gross morphological features. Using specific and easily recognizable landmarks, these gross phases are further subdivided into a series of stages which are compiled into a normal table of development. Such a table has been worked out for *Xenopus* in fine detail. Figure 1.1 gives an overview of the timing of development, and of the different phases and stages.

At fertilization, which is often regarded as the onset of development, the egg has already passed through the long preparatory phase of oogenesis from which the oocyte emerges. Germ cell development is already underway in the early embryonic phases of the mother and it takes many months before the oocyte is fully developed. Both intracellular synthesis and transport from the outside contribute to the growth of the oocyte, which vastly increases in size. The accumulated contents provides the material from which the embryo forms.

A hint of cell polarity is already visible in the earliest phase of oogenesis. This polarity becomes a characteristic feature which dominates the morphology of the oocyte and the egg and later acts as one reference coordinate for early embryogenesis. All morphological features of the oocyte are arranged in radial symmetry around the axis of this polarity. In addition, a number of other structural traits of the oocyte are recognizably directed toward the subsequent development.

A hormone triggers the processes of oocyte maturation. Within a few hours, during which dramatic changes in intracellular organization take place, the oocyte is driven into the meiotic divisions. The first polar body is extruded, and the egg is arrested in the second meiotic metaphase. The egg integument is completed when the egg is released from the mother's body during spawning. The egg is ready for fertilization.

Fertilization triggers the activation reaction by which further development is initiated. A change in the plasma membrane properties and a reorganization of the integument ensures that the egg receives only a single sperm nucleus. The site of sperm entry introduces into the otherwise radially symmetrical system an element of asymmetry. This is later elaborated to become the second reference coordinate completing the primitive axial system along which the early phases of embryogenesis are organized. Bilateral symmetry is established in this way. The second meiotic division is completed and the maternal and paternal pronuclei fuse during karyogamy.

The zygote enters the phase of rapid and synchronous cleavage divisions, which are driven by an oscil-

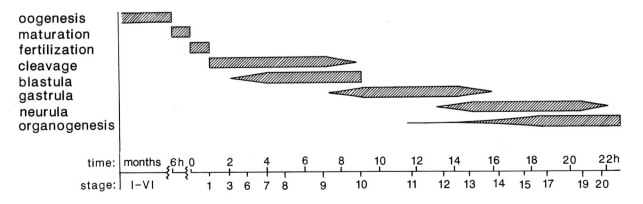

Fig. 1.1. Stages and phases of *Xenopus* development and their timing at 23 °C

3

lating biochemical system acting autonomously in the different regions of the egg. The important morphogenetic events of this phase are the emergence of cells of different sizes, and the generation of apical epithelial junctions which connect the cells of the outer layer. The inner cells which do not participate in junction formation are thereby differentiated from the outer cells. Epithelium formation allows the establishment of physiological ionic conditions within the embryo. Internally, the blastocoel forms as the first prominent extracellular space.

During the cleavage phase the blastula emerges as a multicellular morphological entity. The different regions of the blastula come to form a mosaic pattern of formative tendencies. The cell populations in the different regions become specified for defined types of behavior which are expressed in the characteristic cell movements and cell rearrangements during the forthcoming gastrulation. The first case of induction is involved in the processes which form this pregastrula pattern.

During the gastrula stages the basic vertebrate body plan is generated. A complex set of morphogenetic movements leads to the formation of the three germ layers. Bilateral symmetry is now a prominent feature as anterior and posterior regions together with dorsal and ventral regions of the body define a new and definite system of body axes.

During the morphogenetic movements the different embryonic cell groups pass rapidly through a series of changes in their environment. Cell contacts, cell density, and probably the composition of the extracellular molecular environment vary continuously as the cells become arranged in a new topological system. During these events cells of different provenance have the opportunity to communicate in multiple inductive interactions which generate the program for the next phases of development.

The pattern within the mesoderm that emerges during gastrulation governs the major events of the neurula phase. By inductive interactions with the mesoderm the ectodermal neural plate is formed, which will be transformed in a further set of morphogenetic movements into the neural tube, the an-lage of the central nervous system. Segmentation of the paraxial mesoderm into the individual somites occurs. The basic body structure emerges more and more clearly.

Further development is not so much guided by "global" events, which encompass and remodel the whole embryonic body, but more by the regional processes of organogenesis which extend far into the feeding tadpole stages.

This subdivision of the developmental process into discrete phases is largely arbitrary, since boundaries cannot be strictly defined. Some of the individual subprocesses extend over several phases, others punctuate the stages more clearly. Thus, the formation of the blastula begins with the appearance of the blastocoel anlage during the first cleavage division; gastrulation movements have already begun in the late blastula phase and continue far into the neurula; somitogenesis has its origin in the gastrula and extends into the tadpole stages. Therefore, phasing and staging is largely an aid to structure our observations and should not be allowed to obscure the fact that the closer the process of development is analyzed, the more it appears as a smooth continuum.

This continuum of development extends through the generations. No single event can logically be chosen as the unequivocal onset of development. We begin the outline of *Xenopus* development quite arbitrarily with the description of the fully developed oocyte.

References

NIEUWKOOP, P. D. & FABER, J. (1967). Normal Table of *Xenopus laevis* (Daudin). 2nd edition. Amsterdam: North-Holland Publ. Co.

DAVIDSON, E. H. (1986). Gene Activity in Early Development. 3rd edition. New York: Academic Press.

GERHART, J. C. (1980). Mechanism regulating pattern formation in the amphibian egg and early embryo. In *Biological Regulation and Development* vol. 2 (ed. R. F. Goldberger), pp. 133-292. New York: Plenum Press.

NIEUWKOOP, P. D., JOHNEN, A. G. & ALBERS, B. (1985). The Epigenetic Nature of Chordate Development. Cambridge: Cambridge University Press.

Chapter 2
The Fully Developed Oocyte

The Ovary

The most prominent and conspicuous organ in the belly cavity of a mature *Xenopus* female is the **ovary**. It appears as a transparent bag of connective tissue harboring thousands of **oocytes**. The ovary is subdivided by constrictions into numerous compartments giving it a branched structure. A closer histological analysis (Fig. 2.1) reveals the quite elaborate internal features of the organ. The ovary is surrounded by the outer ovarian epithelium of ciliated cells, which is in actuality part of the visceral peritoneum. It is underlain by the **theca**, a connective tissue layer rich in extracellular matrix which surrounds fibroblastic cells and blood vessels. The inner border of the ovary wall is formed by the inner ovarian epithelium. Oocytes of different developmental stages are located within the theca layer. When the oocytes increase in size, the inner epithelium bulges out and the individual follicles form. A sheet of **follicle cells** surrounds each oocyte, separating it from the theca. An acellular layer of matrix is positioned between the follicle cells and the oocyte membrane; this layer is termed the **vitelline membrane**, or vitelline envelope.

The oocytes can easily be removed from the ovarian tissue for experimental studies, either by dissection or by collagenase treatment. As the size of the oocytes reflects their developmental age, defined size classes can be used to obtain data on the changes of certain parameters during oocyte development. By convention, six stages of oocyte development have been defined using size and other external criteria.

Before discussing the events of oogenesis, a description of the end product of this process, which is the fully grown stage VI oocyte, is required.

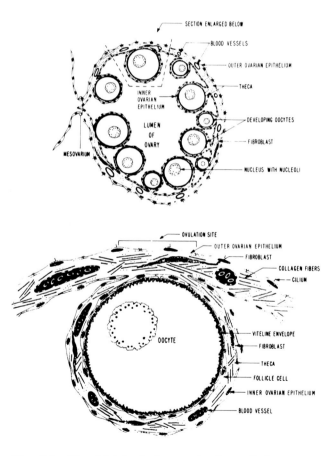

Fig. 2.1. The histological organization of the ovary. (Dumont and Brummet 1978)

The Stage VI Oocyte

The most salient feature of this cell is its vast size: it is a sphere of 1.3 mm in diameter with a volume of 1 µl. The oocyte needs to be this large in order to meet the requirements for providing the material and structural basis for subsequent development. Up to the swimming tadpole stage, when feeding starts, the embryo has to live on the resources accumulated in the oocyte. In addition to the required nutritive supply, the oocyte contains numerous devices and structural features which are needed in embryogenesis. The installation of these features poses extraordinary demands on the developing oocyte, which have been met by a number of specializations unique to the oogenetic cell line. The microscope analysis of a stage VI oocyte reveals some of these features (PLATE 1).

5

Polarity

A pigment pattern provides the oocyte with features of a radially symmetrical body with a distinct polarity. The **animal hemisphere** is dark brown; the **vegetal hemisphere** is only weakly pigmented. The axis of symmetry passes through the animal and the vegetal pole. The two hemispheres are separated by an unpigmented **equatorial belt**. Internally, the excentric position of the nucleus and the structure and staining pattern of the cytoplasm are the most conspicuous expression of the radially symmetrical and polar topology which is manifest in many further details to be described below. The inherent polarity of the arrangement of cellular components is preserved during the subsequent maturation of the oocyte to the ultimate fertilizable egg. It will have a major influence on the emergence of the embryonic structures. In fact, the axis of polarity serves as one coordinate of the geometrical system in which early embryogenesis is organized.

The Nucleus

The nucleus of the oocyte has such an extraordinary appearance that it received a special name in the classical period of embryology, the "**germinal vesicle**", a term still commonly in use. The oocyte nucleus is about 10^5 times larger than that of a normal somatic tissue cell. It is filled with the rather homogeneous **nucleoplasm** in which **chromosomes** and numerous **extranucleoli** are embedded. Although the nucleoplasm appears uniformly stained and evenly distributed within the nucleus, the typical central location of the chromosomes and extranucleoli might indicate that within the nucleoplasm there is a cryptic spatial structure, the nature of which has yet to be elucidated.

The nucleoplasm has been extensively studied. It harbors a complex mixture of proteins, many of which are later refound in the nuclei of the early embryo. It therefore seems likely that the nucleoplasm of the oocyte represents the maternal store of nuclear proteins, which are later required to generate functional nuclei in the embryo. In fact, the germinal vesicle has been found to contain histones, RNA polymerases, and DNA polymerases, each in sufficient amounts to supply several thousand somatic nuclei. Certain acidic proteins (e.g. nucleoplasmin) are present in the germinal vesicle in high concentration. They are able to bind histones, are required for nucleosome assembly during cleavage, and may act as carriers for the transport of histones from the cytoplasm to the nucleus.

A stage VI oocyte contains some 10^{12} ribosomes, but the genome provides only 1800 templates for the synthesis of ribosomal RNA, by far not enough to achieve a rate of rRNA synthesis sufficient to fill the ribosomal store in the time available during oogenesis. This problem has been solved by a process specific to the oocyte: ribosomal RNA genes are amplified some 1500-fold and incorporated into 500 - 2500 extranucleoli. Some of these are seen in the section displayed in PLATE 1.

To achieve a similarly high synthetic rate of the ribosomal 5S RNA another regulatory principle is used: The haploid *Xenopus* genome contains 20 000 5S rRNA genes plus an additional subset of 400 genes with a slightly altered nucleotide sequence. This difference in base sequence results in a difference in affinity of the 5S rRNA genes for the transcription factor TFIIIA. A high concentration of this transcription factor in the oocyte nucleus ensures that both classes of genes are transcribed, whereas in somatic cells, due to their low concentration of TFIIIA, only the second class of genes is active.

Like every cell prior to mitosis the oocyte contains four times the haploid complement of DNA. Yet, this amount of chromatin has to serve a cytoplasm some 10^5- to 10^6-fold the volume of a common somatic cell. As an adaptation to this problem the chromosomes have assumed the well-known lampbrush configuration. They probably represent chromosomes in a state of extraordinarily high activity, with the transcribed regions being fully extended and looping out from the chromosome axis. About 30% of the total DNA sequences are transcribed in these lampbrush chromosomes. Calculations indicate that the high rate of transcription on these chromosomes is just sufficient to maintain the messenger RNA pool at a steady state. In fact, in the stage VI oocytes, the chromosomal loops have already retracted considerably, as compared to earlier stages of oogenesis, and the chromosomes appear quite condensed.

These three examples of transcription in oocytes impressively demonstrate various means for the solution of the same problem, i.e., to achieve a high rate of RNA synthesis.

The nucleus is surrounded by the **nuclear envelope**. In accordance with the high synthetic activity of the nucleus, pore complexes are inserted into the envelope at an unusually high density to allow smooth molecular trafficking. The lobed appearance of the envelope is typical for the oocyte and is probably brought about by the structure of the nuclear lamina, a protein sheet of cytoskeletal nature underlying the lipid bilayer of the nuclear envelope. An oocyte-specific isoform of the lamin protein family is the only constituent polypeptide. It is functional in the oocyte, and at the same time forms the maternal pool, which will later be used in the formation of the early embryonic nuclear envelopes.

The blue basophilic staining on the lateral sides of the nucleus, which is always observed with the histological procedure used in PLATE 1, indicates that the envelope is not homogeneous over the whole surface of the nucleus, and that its features are aligned with the cell's symmetry. As the staining extends a short distance into the lateral cytoplasm, one might speculate that we are looking at sites of preferential nucleocytoplasmic exchange. This suggestion needs to be substantiated.

The Cytoplasm

The most conspicuous feature of the cytoplasm is its high content of **yolk platelets**. The platelets consist of lipo-glyco-phosphoprotein packed in a paracrystalline fashion within a lipid membrane envelope. These platelets serve as "survival packages" for the future embryonic cells and allow them to retain nutritional autonomy for a long time. Yolk protein constitutes up to 80% of the total protein of the oocyte.

The size of the yolk platelets and their distribution within the cytoplasm is not homogeneous. The yolk pattern is an eye-catching expression of the radially symmetrical polarity of the oocyte. The yolk content of the cytoplasm is relatively low in the upper animal hemisphere and increases in a graded fashion, reaching a maximum in the vegetal region. The animal hemisphere harbors mainly small yolk platelets, which are arranged in clusters separated by yolk-free "channels" radiating from the nuclear region to the periphery. These **radii** are rich in intermediate filaments; they stain with antivimentin antibodies, and are probably an overt expression of a more intricate general structuring of the cytoplasm by the cytoskeleton. Isolated yolk platelets are found to be surrounded by a net of actin filaments.

As one moves in the vegetal direction, the yolk platelets increase in size, the largest ones being located at the vegetal margin. The central region of the cytoplasm is separated from the outer region by an **intracytoplasmic boundary** of differential staining, which is continuous with the above mentioned lateral edges of the nucleus. This boundary is revealed with various staining methods; its function and special molecular characteristics are unknown. Outside this boundary small yolk platelets are intermingled with larger ones. This yolk pattern will become better understood when the process of vitellogenesis during oogenesis is discussed in more detail.

The yolk pattern seems to bear some intriguing relation to the subsequent embryogenesis. The yellowish-stained vegetal region poor in cytoplasm between the yolk platelets will later form most of the endodermal yolk mass. This region will be shifted to the interior of the embryo during gastrulation and eventually end up in the intestinal lumen, where it will be digested and serve as the primary food supply of the swimming tadpole. The more bluish-stained animal and equatorial regions are richer in cytoplasm. They will give rise to most of those cells from which the embryo proper is formed. An inkling of the future embryonic role of these regions is thus apparent.

A number of the molecular characteristics of the cytoplasm are of relevance to processes of embryogenesis. Although the oocyte is very active in protein synthesis, only about 2% of the ribosomes are bound to mRNA and are thus active in translation. The remainder forms a store that will function later. Similarly, only about 20% of the mRNA is active in translation, the remainder is bound to a specific set of proteins to form inactive RNP particles, again in preparation for forthcoming events. The complexity of the mRNA is high; some 20 000 different species are thought to reside in the oocyte. [The cytoplasmic poly(A) RNA in oocytes is remarkable, as a large fraction of it contains middle repitive sequences, a feature otherwise found only in nuclear poly(A) RNA. Its function in the oocyte has remained a long-standing enigma.]

The oocyte cytoplasm has means to localize certain mRNAs at specific sites. For example, one mRNA species, vg-1, is exclusively found in the subcortical cytoplasm of the vegetal half. The localization of this RNA is thought to be important for future development.

The Cortex

A border zone, from which the yolk platelets are excluded, extends from the **plasma membrane** a few microns into the interior. This **cortex** is not a well-defined structure, as no clear border separates it from the underlying cytoplasm. A prominent character of the cortex is its relative rigidity and tensile strength which contributes to the mechanical stability of the cell. This allows the mechanical isolation of the cortex or pieces of it. Biochemical analysis reveals a complex composition. The most prominent cytoskeletal elements are actin fibers which may confer to the cortical region the ability to contract, a feature which is required in the early phases after fertilization. Cytokeratin is arranged in the cortex in a specific pattern. In the vegetal hemisphere it forms a highly regular network, whereas in the animal half it is arranged in a more irregular fashion.

Some organelles are specifically localized within the cortical region, the most conspicuous ones are the **pigment granules**. They consist of packed membranous elements, heavily loaded with melanin. The pigment granule density is closely correlated with the oocyte polarity, giving to the oocyte the typical external pigmentation pattern. One may only speculate on the function of this pigment pattern. It is almost certainly an ecological adaptation, serving either to protect the egg and the embryo against damaging light, or to camouflage them against predators. In either case, the pigment is required on the body surface of the embryo. As the epidermis covering the body of the future embryo is derived from the heavily pigmented animal peripheral region of the egg, the pigment distribution shows again how the structural organization of the oocyte is directed toward forthcoming events.

Cortical granules are a second kind of organelle typical for the cortex. They may be recognized in favorable regions of PLATE 1 using a magnifying lens (see also PLATES 3G; 9H). A dense layer of blue-stained granules about 2 μm in diameter lines the plasma membrane. They are membrane-surrounded vesicles, which are filled with a mixture of glycoproteins ready to be exocytosed to the outside at fertilization. The cortical granules of the animal and vegetal region differ somewhat in size, emphasizing that the cell polarity is expressed in many details.

The cortical zone extends into numerous microvilli, which penetrate the vitelline layer, interdigitate, and make contact via gap junctions with the microvilli of the cells of the **follicle layer** which surrounds the oocyte. It would be of much interest to learn what function these contacts serve.

The Vitelline Layer

A layer of extracellular matrix is localized in the oocyte-follicle cell interphase. This **vitelline membrane** serves specialized functions in the process of fertilization and early embryogenesis. Scanning electron microscopy reveals a mat consisting of loosely packed 4 - 7 nm filaments, punctuated by large pores through which the microvillar contacts between the oocyte and the follicle cells are established. The molecular structure of the vitelline membrane is not precisely known, but it contains several glycosylated polypeptides which are not found elsewhere in extracellular matrix material.

The Oocyte as an Experimental Tool

Due to their vast size, oocytes may easily be microinjected with various materials to be assayed for biological activity. They respond upon injection of DNA into the germinal vesicle by specific transcription; upon injection of mRNA into the cytoplasm by synthesis of the corresponding proteins. Injected proteins find their way to specific intracellular locations; for example, if nuclear proteins are injected into the cytoplasm, they will enter the nucleus. Membrane proteins, translated from injected mRNA will insert into the membrane. These experiments are performed to investigate the molecular and cellular biology of the oocyte, but much more frequently to analyze the biological activity of the injected molecules, the oocyte thereby being used as a "living test tube".

A useful compilation of molecular data on the stage VI oocyte is given in Table 2.1.

References

See references to Chapter 3 (pp. 13, 14).

Table 2.1. Composition of a fully grown *Xenopus* oocyte without follicle cells. Total volume, 1 μl; yolk-free volume, 0.5 μl; GV volume, 40 nl

Component	Weight	Number of components	% of total in cytoplasm
DNA			
Chromosomal	12 pg	–	None
Nucleolar (rDNA)	25 pg	2×10^6 rDNA repeats	None
Mitochondrial	4000 pg	$\sim 10^8$ Genomes	100
RNA			
Ribosomal	5 μg	10^{12} Ribosomes	99
5S	60 ng	10^{12}	99
tRNA	60 ng	1.5×10^{12}	99
snRNA U1	0.07 ng	8×10^8	99
PolyA + RNA	80 ng	5×10^{10} (if 2500 bases long)	90
Ribosomal protein mRNA	10 ng	2×10^{10}	–
Actin mRNA	$\sim$ 1 ng	5×10^8	–
Heat-shock 70 mRNA	0.004 ng	10^6	–
Protein			
Yolk	250 μg	–	100
Non-yolk	25 μg	5×10^{14} (30 K protein)	90
Histones	140 ng	5×10^{12}	50
Nucleoplasmin	250 ng	5×10^{12}	98
RNA polymerase I and II		$\sim 10^5 \times$ Somatic cell	–
RNA polymerase III		$5 \times 10^5 \times$ Somatic cell	–
Precursors			
dTTP	10 pmol	–	–
rGTP	250 pmol	–	–
Methionine	40 pmol	–	–

(After Gurdon and Wakefield 1986)

Chapter 3
Oogenesis

The features of the fully developed oocyte, which were described in the preceding chapter, arise according to a well-patterned schedule. Many of them are of fundamental importance for future embryogenesis. Their emergence demonstrates how the processes of oogenesis are already directed toward the development of the new individual. Oogenesis is an integral part of the epigenetic process which generates the embryo.

The Oogonial Stages

The origin of the oocyte can be traced back to the early developmental stages of the mother. At day 4 of development primordial germ cells, which were segregated as a specialized cell line during the earliest embryonic phases, invade the as yet sexually undifferentiated gonads and by day 8, 25 - 30 of these cells have settled in the gonadal anlage. During the next 2.5 weeks the cells remain quiescent.

In the early stages primordial germ cells still have the potency to differentiate into either male or female gametes. The decision as to which pathway they take depends on the sexual type of the surrounding soma and not on their own chromosome constitution. If male primordial germ cells are transplanted into a female embryo, oocytes with a male set of chromosomes are formed and, vice versa, spermatocytes with a female set of chromosomes may be produced by the reverse manipulation.

At 3 weeks of age the gonads become sexually differentiated and the primordial germ cells resume multiplication. If female, they are now termed **primary oogonia**. Multiplication is asynchronous and slow. Primary oogonia are larger than the somatic cells of the surrounding gonad and therefore easily discerned (PLATE 2A,B). Their nucleus is lobed and irregular in shape, with the variably condensed chromatin unevenly distributed and conspicuous nucleoli.

By the age of 4 weeks after fertilization pairs of oogonia coupled together by an intercellular bridge are found in the young ovary. This feature classifies them as **secondary oogonia**. The bridge is maintained while these cells undergo three further divisions which occur in synchrony, probably due to their cytoplasmic coupling (PLATE 2C).

The Early Meiotic Prophase

The daughters of one founder primary oogonium eventually form a nest of 16 pear-shaped cells, with their bridge-connected tips lying at the center of the nest. After the last division one further round of DNA replication reconstitutes their 4C DNA content and cell division is arrested for the next months. It is resumed at maturation, after the oocyte has undergone a long period of development and intracellular patterning.

The young oocytes remain connected by cytoplasmic bridges throughout the next stages of the meiotic prophase which occur in perfect synchrony within one nest. Sections through young ovaries reveal the whole sequence of the meiotic prophase stages

Table 3.1. Stages of the growing oocytes

Stage	I	II	III	IV	V	VI
Size [μm]	50−300	300−450	450−600	600−1000	1000−1200	1200−1300
Appearance	Transparent	Opaque, white	Light brown	Animal-vegetal difference in pigmentation	Hemispheres clearly delineated	Unpigmented equatorial belt

(After Dumont 1972)

(Fig. 3.4). At **leptotene** the nucleus has lost its lobed appearance and the chromatin is more condensed (PLATE 2E). **Synaptonemal complexes** form during zygotene. The **pachytene** stage is characterized by the maximal expression of the synaptonemal complexes, abutting the nuclear envelope nearest the center of the nest. Their arrangement reflects the familiar bouquet formation of the paired homologues (PLATE 2F).

At late pachytene, the cells of a nest become separated from one another. The chromosomes assume the **lampbrush configuration** as the cells pass into the **diplotene** stage (PLATES 2G,H; 9A,B). The young oocytes now become surrounded by follicle cells. They remain in diplotene until the meiotic divisions are completed during oocyte maturation, by which time the oocyte has increased in diameter from 20 μm to 1.3 mm, corresponding to a 3×10^5-fold increase in volume. The length of the growth period depends on the hormonal condition of the mother and may last for several months. External criteria are used to define the stages of the growing diplotene oocytes (Table 3.1).

The Growing Oocyte

We will now consider some characteristic features of the oocyte as they emerge during oogenesis, with emphasis on those events which are overtly expressed in the morphology of the growing oocytes (PLATES 2; 3).

Extranucleoli and Ribosomal RNA Synthesis

In order to meet the demands of the oocyte and the embryo, for large amounts of ribosomes, rRNA genes are amplified during oogenesis and incorporated into numerous extranucleoli.

Already in the oogonial stage, well before a recognizable sexual differentiation of the germ cells has occurred, an enigmatic and abortive prelude of rDNA amplification is observed. The cells are found to contain a variable number of (up to 9) nucleoli and the amount of rDNA has increased 5–40 times in the individual gonia. During the transition into the meiotic prophase this extra rDNA seems to be lost from the cells.

Amplification is resumed at zygotene. At pachytene the original nucleoli are localized in a chromatin-free region within the nucleus called the **nuclear cap** (PLATE 2F). This region is very active in rDNA synthesis and contains abundant rDNA as revealed by thymidine labeling and in situ hybridization. At early diplotene the amplified DNA becomes organized into extranucleoli, the number of which eventually reaches 500–2500 per nucleus. They are first seen in the original nuclear cap region and are later shifted toward the periphery of the nucleus until they become scattered throughout the nucleoplasm. In oocytes at stages above IV the number of extranucleoli decreases, probably due to fusion as indicated by their heterogeneity in size (PLATES 3A–E; 9A–C).

Ribosomal RNA synthesis from the amplified DNA starts at stage II and might reach the maximal theoretical rate for the given number of rRNA genes at stages III–IV. Some 3×10^5 rRNA molecules/sec are being synthesized as compared to 10–100/sec in somatic cells. There is a continuous accumulation of rRNA during the whole period of oogenesis. The rate of transcription decreases in stage VI oocytes but, depending on the hormonal conditions in the female, up to half of the maximal rate may be retained.

The Chromosomes and Poly(A) RNA Synthesis

During the earlier meiotic prophases the chromosomes exhibit a rather condensed structure. They begin to unfold visibly into the familiar lampbrush configuration at the early diplotene of stage I and assume their maximal extension at stages I–III, whereafter the lampbrush loops begin to retract. At stages V and VI the chromosomes appear as quite condensed strands in the light microscope. PLATE 9 depicts these features best.

The lampbrush state of the chromosomes indicates maximal transcriptional activity. In fact, stage II oocytes begin to accumulate large amounts of poly(A) RNA, and at stage III the full complement of this RNA is already present in the oocytes. Further transcriptional activity is apparently solely required to counterbalance poly(A) RNA degradation. The total amount of the poly(A) RNA is kept constant during stages III–VI in this way.

There is no recognizable differential regulation of gene activity in these stages of oogenesis. If assayed for specific mRNA sequences their pattern of accumulation much reflects that of the total poly(A) RNA. Most of the newly accumulated poly(A) RNA is stored in the form of inactive RNP particles. Beginning at stage II, mRNA is increasingly recruited from the particles to participate in protein synthesis, which continuously rises during the next stages of oogenesis. The mRNA recruitment is continued into early embryogenesis until at midblastula the maternal store of mRNA begins to run low and transcription provides new templates for further protein synthesis.

Mitochondria

The fully developed oocyte contains some 10^5 times more mitochondria than a "normal" somatic cell, such that the amount of mitochondrial DNA exceeds that of the chromosomal DNA by a factor of 300–400. This large number of mitochondria is produced throughout oogenesis. They become temporarily aggregated into conspicuous structures which are a prominent feature of young oocytes. The staining method chosen in PLATES 2 and 3 reveals the **mitochondrial aggregates** with a characteristic reddish color.

The mitochondrial aggregate is most obvious in stage I oocytes as a single spherical body adjacent to the nuclear membrane (PLATES 2H; 3A). This structure is a feature common to the oocytes of many different species and has such an extraordinary appearance that it has been described independently several times and endowed with a number of names. It is cited in the literature as the Balbiani body, the mitochondrial cloud, the mitochondrial aggregate, the mitochondrial mass, or the yolk nucleus.

Electron microscopy of this structure reveals a close aggregate of mitochondria embedded in an electron-dense granular material (mitochondrial cement), together with electron-dense particles (nuage), Golgi structures, and cytoskeletal elements.

Ultrastructural studies further indicate that the Balbiani body has its origin in mitochondrial aggregates already present in the primordial germ cells; the aggregates are a common feature of all early stages of oogenesis (PLATE 2). Concomitant with the growth of the diplotene oocyte, the mitochondrial aggregate increases in size (PLATES 2F,G,H; 3A).

At stage II, the Balbiani body decays into numerous smaller fragments which segregate into two populations (PLATE 3B,C). One portion of the fragments becomes localized to the perinuclear region from where the mitochondria are eventually distributed throughout the cytoplasm. The other portion of the fragments shifts in a remarkably polarized movement toward the cortex of one side of the oocyte, where it becomes deposited and may be identified throughout the further stages of oogenesis (Fig. 3.1).

The functional significance of the Balbiani body is not well understood. Since mitochondria are produced throughout oogenesis, their association with the Balbiani body does not seem to be a prerequisite for their replication, though a high rate of mitochondrial DNA synthesis is found within the body. Possibly, the Balbiani body and the sophisticated way in which it fragments serve the function of distributing mitochondria adequately into all cytoplasmic regions of the oocyte.

As will be described later, the cortical population of Balbiani body fragments will become included into the primordial germ cells of the developing embryo. The directed movement of the fragments may serve to ensure a sufficient allocation of mitochondria to these cells. The inclusion of the Balbiani body-derived material into the prospective primordial germ cells has often given rise to considerations that it harbors some as yet to be detected "germ cell determinants". The debate on this topic is not closed.

Vitellogenesis

When the growing oocyte has reached a size of 400 μm in diameter at stage III, the period of vitellogenesis commences, during which large amounts of yolk appear in the oocyte. The yolk protein precursor vitellogenin, which is produced in the liver and released into the blood stream, is collected from the blood by receptors on the oocyte surface and transported through the oocyte membrane by receptor-mediated endocytosis. Most of the increase in oocyte size during this final period of oogenesis is accounted for by the uptake of yolk protein, which eventually makes up 80% of the total oocyte protein.

In vitro studies have indicated that the rate of oocyte growth in the vitellogenic stages depends critically on the availability of vitellogenin in the surrounding medium. Since the synthesis of this protein in the liver is under hormonal control, the rate of oocyte growth is influenced by the hormonal system of the mother as well. In young animals, a period of 1−1.5 years is required to produce fully developed oocytes. In gonadotropin stimulated females vitellogenesis requires only approximately 2 months.

As a result of the endocytosis, vesicles containing vitellogenin appear beneath the oocyte surface. They fuse into "transitional yolk bodies" of various sizes. Within these bodies vitellogenin is cleaved into the yolk proteins, phosvitin and lipovitellin, which are deposited in a paracrystalline fashion. Yolk platelets are formed from these bodies by fusion, and the growth of the platelets continues as further transitional yolk bodies are apposed to them. Production of new platelets and the growth of the individual platelets continues throughout vitellogenesis (Fig. 3.2). Accordingly, the size of the largest yolk platelets correlates with the age of the oocyte.

Some of these features show up in the illustrations of PLATE 3. At the beginning of vitellogenesis, the oocyte contains **lipid deposits** which are later seen in close association with yolk, until they disappear completely from oocytes of the late stages (PLATE 3B,C,D). Very small yolk bodies are seen in the cortex of young vitellogenic oocytes (PLATE 3C), with advancing age of the oocytes their yolk platelets increase in size. At stage IV the

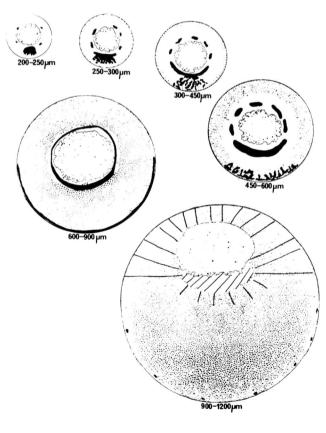

Fig. 3.1. Distribution of mitochondrial aggregates during the vitellogenic phase of oogenesis. (Tourte et al. 1984)

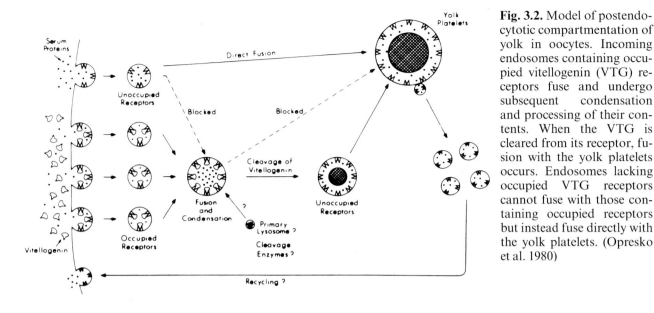

Fig. 3.2. Model of postendocytotic compartmentation of yolk in oocytes. Incoming endosomes containing occupied vitellogenin (VTG) receptors fuse and undergo subsequent condensation and processing of their contents. When the VTG is cleared from its receptor, fusion with the yolk platelets occurs. Endosomes lacking occupied VTG receptors cannot fuse with those containing occupied receptors but instead fuse directly with the yolk platelets. (Opresko et al. 1980)

selectivity of the cortical granule movement toward the surface is indicated by the countertraffic of the newly formed yolk platelets which move simultaneously inwards.

Pigment granules begin to be deposited in the cortex of oocytes at stage III. Initially, the pigment is evenly distributed over the whole cortex. During stage IV the animal-vegetal polarity becomes expressed in the pigment pattern, with the vegetal cortex being less pigmented than the animal cortex. PLATE 3E gives an indication of how this may be brought about: the whole cortical zone becomes polarized in stage IV oocytes, the vegetal cortex is thinned, possibly by stretching, while the cortical region in the animal half does not undergo thinning and remains much thicker. Pigment granules may thus become unevenly distributed. Eventually, pigment granules and cortical granules form two separate layers at the oocyte surface: the cortical granules bordering the plasma membrane and the pigment occupying a position deeper in the cortex.

size of the yolk platelets forms a gradient along the radius of the cell, the larger platelets being located more centrally. Such observations imply that yolk is moved during its formation from the surface into the interior of the growing oocyte.

The size distribution of the yolk platelets in the fully grown oocyte forms a distinct pattern along the animal-vegetal axis. Recent experiments have elucidated the generation of this pattern.

If vitellogenin, labeled with a fluorescent ligand, is injected into the blood stream of an adult female, uptake of the label by the oocytes occurs within a limited period of time. In such "pulse-labeled" oocytes growth of the yolk platelets and their transport within the oocyte may be traced by inspection of sections from oocytes at different stages and at different times after introduction of the labeled yolk protein. It turns out that, in addition to the centripetal migration of the yolk platelets, a second vector of movement, which is aligned with the polarity of the cell, contributes to the final pattern. Yolk from the animal hemisphere is transported into the vegetal half. As a result, a gradient of yolk density is established in the animal-vegetal direction. Older

and larger platelets are abundant in the vegetal half, whereas the animal half harbors mainly smaller and younger platelets. Figure 3.3 depicts the emergence of the yolk pattern during vitellogenesis schematically. The movement of the yolk during oocyte growth is most probably a function of the cytoskeleton. The radii found in the animal half of stage V and VI oocytes may be a manifestation of this intracellular transport system. The stage VI oocyte may be called the postvitellogenic oocyte. This cell shows only little endocytotic activity, and yolk accumulation has ceased.

The Cortex

Two types of organelles typical for the cortex are formed during the later phases of oogenesis: the cortical granules and the pigment granules.

Cortical granules are first found in the peripheral cytoplasm of stage II oocytes. They move toward the surface, as the oocyte increases in size, and finally become aligned in a dense layer underneath the plasma membrane (PLATES 3F,G; 9H). The

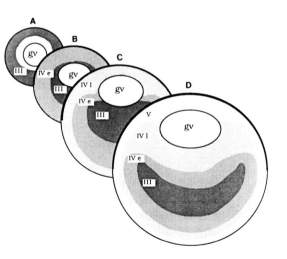

Fig. 3.3. Redistribution of yolk platelets along the animal-vegetal axis during vitellogenesis. **A** Late stage III oocyte; **B** early stage IV oocyte; **C** late stage IV/early stage V oocyte; **D** late stage V oocyte. The intensity of *shading* indicates the relative age of the yolk platelets. The *Roman numerals* indicate the oocyte stage at which the yolk has been pinocytosed. (Danilchik and Gerhart 1987)

The Vitelline Membrane

When the follicle layer forms at stage I, the oocyte surface contacts the follicle cells via microvilli. The acellular vitelline membrane begins to appear in the spaces between the microvilli at stage III.

The Origin of the Animal-Vegetal Polarity

The origin of the oocyte polarity cannot be attributed to a determinative influence of external cues. The oocytes are oriented in the ovary at random with respect to gravity. Likewise, the orientation of the oocyte axis bears no relation to the ovarian walls or blood vessels. Influences of such parameters on the establishment of the oocyte axis are therefore unlikely. A determinative influence of the follicle cells can be excluded since polarity is already expressed when the layer forms.

There are, on the other hand, strong arguments in favor of the notion that the axis forms autonomously in the oocyte. Formally, an axis of polarity is given in each cell by the line which passes through the nucleus and the centrosome. Apparently, it is this axis of the oogonium which is elaborated to form the conspicuous animal-vegetal polarity of the oocyte. Starting from the oogonium, several morphological features express the axial organization during the various stages of oocyte development, such that the cell polarity may be followed throughout oogenesis (Fig. 3.4).

The secondary oogonia are pear-shaped and exhibit a distinct polar arrangement of the organelles. Golgi structures are localized toward the tip of the cell. The nucleus is positioned in the main body of the cell. The mitochondrial mass, which occupies a position between the nucleus and the tip of the cell, harbors the centriole. These features define an axis of polarity in the oogonia. During the next stages the nuclear differentiations in the meiotic prophase are also arranged according to this polarity. The synaptonemal complexes abut the nuclear membrane next to the mitochondrial mass, and in

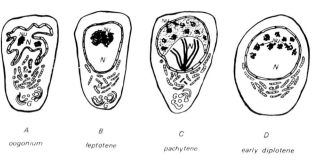

A	*B*	*C*	*D*
oogonium	leptotene	pachytene	early diplotene

Fig. 3.4. Schematic representation of the evolution of nucleus, mitochondria, and Golgi apparatus during early oogenesis, with regard to a hypothetical axis. Relative positions of the nucleus (N), nucleoli (Nu), mitochondria (M), and Golgi apparatus (G) remain the same from oogonium to diplotene stage. (Tourte et al. 1981)

pachytene and early diplotene the cap structure is formed in the nuclear region opposite the mitochondrial mass. At stage II the behavior of the mitochondrial mass during its fragmentation gives a clear indication of the oocyte polarity. The cortical population of fragments migrates toward the future vegetal pole. Later, the uneven distribution of yolk platelets becomes the most obvious manifestation of the polarity. During stage IV the asymmetric thinning of the cortex results in an uneven distribution of the pigment granules. As a consequence, polarity becomes externally visible. Internally, the asymmetric transport of yolk from the animal to the vegetal hemisphere may contribute to the dislocation of the nucleus into the animal hemisphere.

It will become obvious in later chapters that orderly embryonic development critically depends on the polar organization of the oocyte. The observations on its emergence demonstrate how oogenesis is from its very beginning part of the developmental process.

References

Reviews

BLACKLER, A. W. (1970). The integrity of the reproductive cell line in the amphibia. In *Curr. Top. Dev. Biol.* **5**, 71-87.

DREYER, C. (1989). Fate and nuclear localization of germinal vesicle proteins during embryogenesis. In *Developmental Biology*, vol. 6 (ed. L. W. Browder), pp. 31-57. New York: Plenum Press.

DREYER, C., WANG, Y. H., WEDLICH, D. & HAUSEN, P. (1983). Oocyte nuclear proteins in the development of *Xenopus*. In *Current Problems in Germ Cell Differentiation*, 7th Symposium of the British Society for Developmental Biology (ed. A. McLaren & C. C. Wylie), pp. 329-351. Cambridge: Cambridge University Press.

DUMONT, J. N. (1972). Oogenesis in *Xenopus laevis* (Daudin). I. Stages of oocyte development in laboratory maintained animals. *J. Morphol.* **136**, 153-180.

DUMONT, J. N. & BRUMMETT, A. R. (1985). Egg envelopes in vertebrates. In *Developmental Biology*, vol.1 (ed. L. W. Browder), pp. 235-258. New York: Plenum Press.

GURDON, J. B. & WAKEFIELD, L. (1986). Microinjection of amphibian oocytes and eggs for the analysis of transcription. In *Microinjection and Organelle Transplantation Techniques* (ed. J. F. Celis, A. Graessmann & A. Loyter), pp. 269-299. London: Academic Press.

HEIKKILA, J. J. (1989). Use of *Xenopus* oocytes to study the expression of cloned genes and translation of messenger RNA. *Biotechnology* **7**, 47-59.

RICHTER, D. J. (1987). Molecular mechanism of translational control during early development of *Xenopus laevis*. In *Translational Regulation of Gene Expression* (ed. J. Ilan), pp. 111-139. New York: Plenum Press.

SMITH, L. D. (1986). Regulation of translation during amphibian oogenesis and oocyte maturation. In *Gametogenesis and the Early Embryo*. 44th Symposium of the Society for Developmental Biology (ed. J. G. Gall), pp. 131-150. New York: Alan R. Liss Inc.

SMITH, L. D. & RICHTER, J. D. (1985). Synthesis, accumulation and utilization of maternal macromolecules during oogenesis and oocyte maturation. In *Biology of Fertilization* (ed. A. Monroy & C. Metz), pp. 141-160. New York: Academic Press.

WALLACE, R. A. (1983). Interactions between somatic cells and the growing oocyte of *Xenopus laevis*. In *Current Problems in Germ Cell Differentiation*, 7th Symposium of the British Society of Developmental Biology (ed. A. McLaren & C. C. Wylie), pp. 285-306. Cambridge: Cambridge University Press.

AL-MUKHTAR, K. A. K. & WEBB, A. C. (1971). An ultrastructural study of primordial germ cells, oogonia and early oocytes in *Xenopus laevis*. *J. Embryol. Exp. Morphol.* **26**, 195-217.

BILLETT, F. S. & ADAM, E. (1976). The structure of the mitochondrial cloud of *Xenopus laevis*. *J. Embryol. Exp. Morphol.* **36**, 697-710.

COGGINS, W. L. (1973). An ultrastructural and radioautographic study of early oogenesis in the toad *Xenopus laevis*. *J. Cell Sci.* **12**, 71-93.

DANILCHIK, M. V. & GERHART, J. C. (1987). Differentiation of the animal-vegetal axis in *Xenopus laevis* oocytes. I. Polarized intracellular translocation of platelets establishes the yolk gradient. *Dev. Biol.* **122**, 101-112.

DUMONT, J. N. & BRUMMETT, A. R. (1978). Oogenesis in *Xenopus laevis* (Daudin). V. Relationships between developing oocytes and their investing follicular tissues. *J. Morphol.* **155**, 73-98.

KALT, M. R. (1973). Ultrastructural observations on the germ line of *Xenopus laevis*. *Z. Zellforsch.* **138**, 41-62.

KALT, M. R. & GALL, J. G. (1974). Observations on early germ cell development and premeiotic ribosomal DNA amplification in *Xenopus laevis*. *J. Cell Biol.* **62**, 460-472.

MIGNOTTE, F., TOURTE, M. & MOUNOLOU, J. C. (1987). Segregation of mitochondria in the cytoplasm of *Xenopus* vitellogenic oocytes. *Biol. Cell.* **60**, 97-102.

OPRESKO, L., WILEY, H. S. & WALLACE, R. A. (1980). Differential postendocytotic compartmentation in *Xenopus laevis* oocytes is mediated by a specifically bound ligand. *Cell* **22**, 47-57.

TOURTE, M., MIGNOTTE, F. & MOUNOLOU, J. C. (1981). Organization and replication activity of the mitochondrial mass of oogonia and previtellogenic oocytes in *Xenopus laevis*. *Dev. Growth Differ.* **23**, 9-21.

TOURTE, M., MIGNOTTE, F. & MOUNOLOU, J. C. (1984). Heterogeneous distribution and replication activity of mitochondria in *Xenopus laevis* oocytes. *Eur. J. Cell Biol.* **34**, 171-178.

Chapter 4
Oocyte Maturation

Under natural conditions, spawning is initiated in a population of frogs by a combination of seasonal influences, conditions of the pond water such as temperature and algal growth, and social cooperation within the population. Gonadotropin is released from the female's pituitary gland triggering the egg-laying response.

In the laboratory these ecological conditions may be circumvented by an injection of gonadotropin into the female's lymphatic system. This induces the complex physiological reaction of spawning, including such diverse phenomena as copulation behavior, the preparation of the oviduct for the production of egg envelope components, and the production of progesterone by the follicle cells. Oocytes are released from their follicles into the peritoneal cavity from where they are transported into the oviduct by ciliary movement. During these events the oocytes perform a series of reactions, collectively known as "oocyte maturation" or "egg maturation". In vitro this reaction may be observed when isolated oocytes are incubated with progesterone.

The Initiation of Oocyte Maturation

During oogenesis cell division occurs only in the oogonial stages. Division is then halted, the cells remain in interphase during the stages of meiotic prophase, which last for several months until the fully grown oocyte has developed. Oocyte maturation now releases this block and the cell is driven into the first meiotic division. The second meiotic division is resumed immediately after completion of the first one, but is arrested in the second metaphase until fertilization initiates further development. Thus oocyte maturation may be viewed, in a first approximation, as that complex of events by which a cell makes its transition from the G_2 period of interphase into the M phase of the cell cycle. This concept stimulated much research on the molecular events of the maturation process, taking oocyte maturation as a model system for studies on the mitotic cycle in general. This view has proven to be very fruitful. Many of the results obtained with oocytes also apply to somatic cells and vice versa results of studies on other systems also apply to oocyte maturation.

The maturation process is triggered by the binding of progesterone to a receptor associated with the oocyte's plasma membrane. Clearly, the hormone acts from the outside, since hormone coupled to polystyrene beads, which do not cross the plasma membrane, is still active, and hormone injected into the oocyte has no effect. These results are somewhat surprising, since steroid hormones are usually known to bind to intracellular receptors that enter the nucleus and act as regulators of transcription.

The morphological effects of this hormonal stimulus, most noticeably the disintegration of the oocyte nucleus (germinal vesicle breakdown, GVBD) and the formation of the maturation spindle, are recognized only after a period of 3−5 h has elapsed. Much of the current research on the mechanism of the maturation process is aimed at the processes which occur during this delay and how the outer signal is transduced and relayed to the intracellular effectors.

A cascade of intracellular events has been monitored after the application of progesterone to oocytes. A transient increase of free Ca^{2+} has been recorded within the first minutes. The level of cyclic AMP and the activity of adenylate cyclase decrease, influencing the activity of cAMP-dependent kinases. A depolarization of the membrane potential can be detected 1 h after the hormone addition accompanied by K^+ efflux and Na^+ influx. The intracellular pH rises at the same time. Phosphorylation of ribosomal protein S6 is then elevated six to eight times and the rate of total protein synthesis increases by a factor of 2−3. Approximately 1 h before GVBD phosphorylation of numerous nonribosomal proteins commences.

Treating oocytes with various drugs can facilitate, inhibit, or induce the maturation process. The nature of these drugs clearly indicates that the activation of the maturation reaction involves well-known second messenger pathways.

The current discussion centers around the question of as to how the observed diverse effects are causally linked. A key link in the chain of events is an autocatalytic process which, once it is triggered, sustains and drives the maturation reaction. A factor indispensable for a successful maturation, the "maturation promoting factor" (MPF), is formed shortly before GVBD from a pool of inactive pro-MPF. Synthesis of an as yet unknown protein is required to initiate this reaction. Once traces of active MPF appear in the cell, further pro-MPF is converted to MPF. An injection of small amounts of cytoplasm containing active MPF into resting oocytes causes them to produce more MPF, which may then be

transferred to another oocyte, and so on. This experiment demonstrates the autocatalysis mentioned above. The early events which normally precede the rise of MPF activity are bypassed by injecting traces of this key molecule, and the injected oocytes undergo normal maturation.

MPF has been purified almost to homogeneity. The fraction contains only two major subunits (cdc-2 and cyclin), one of which becomes phosphorylated in the presence of ATP. It is therefore likely that the MPF has kinase activity and amplifies this activity by autophosphorylation or by the inactivation of an enzyme system that prevents the conversion of inactive pro-MPF to MPF.

Apparently, pro-MPF is held inactive in the resting oocyte by the delicate balance of a system of different protein kinases and their regulators. Any destabilization of this balance by experimentation may quite unpredictably trigger the autocatalytic reaction. It is therefore difficult to be certain whether any given experimental manipulation, which induces maturation, does in fact affect a process in the normal, physiological chain of reactions. In spite of such problems, the signal transduction pathway is being unraveled and flow diagram schemes can be proposed, one of which is depicted in Fig. 4.1.

The activation of MPF drives the cell into the first meiotic division which is completed by the formation of the first **polar body**. The second meiotic division is initiated but arrested at metaphase. This condition becomes stabilized by a further component of the system, the cytostatic factor (CSF), until the block is released after fertilization.

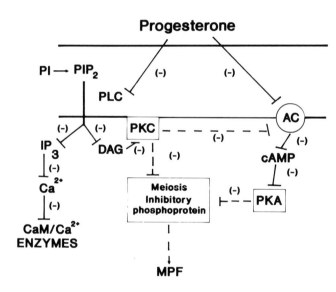

Fig. 4.1. Model depicting the roles of both protein kinase A (*PKA*) and protein kinase C (*PKC*) in the induction of oocyte maturation. Progesterone acts at the oocyte membrane to reduce both adenylate cyclase (*AC*) activity and that of the phosphodiesterase (*PLC*) which cleaves phosphatidylinositol 4,5-biphosphate (*PIP$_2$*). Reduction in AC activity leads to decreased PKA activity. Decreased PLC activity lowers the level of inositol trisphosphate (*IP$_3$*) and diacylglycerol (*DAG*). Decreased DAG is postulated to inactivate PKC, resulting in dephosphorylation of the putative inhibitory phosphoprotein and/or reducing *cAMP* levels via action on AC. *Dashed lines* refer to reactions which are not yet documented in the oocyte. (Smith 1989)

sion of the structural transformation of an oocyte being driven into the first meiotic division. The illustrations induce us to contemplate on how remote the results on the molecular level still are from giving a satisfying explanation of these coordinated movements and structural changes.

All the changes are related to the animal-vegetal polarity of the oocyte, the radial symmetry of which is in principle preserved, though the transient morphological patterns are not rigidly reproduced in all oocytes. There is always a certain individual variation, which may result in some deviation from radial symmetry. Apparently, this variation has no effect on normal embryogenesis.

The first obvious feature, which seems to initiate the cascade of structural changes, is the emergence of a **yolk-free zone** at the basal side of the nucleus (PLATE 4). Under favorable conditions **fascicles of fibers** may be observed being aligned tangentially to the nuclear envelope within this area (PLATE 9D). The fibers have been shown to contain microtubules in high amounts. Apparently, a giant microtubular organization center is being established beneath the nucleus. Incidentally, this is the site within the cell, where the centrosome, a microtubular organization center common to all somatic cells, disappeared after the last mitotic division in the oogonial stage. This finding represents an interesting case of continuity of a cytoplasmic structure over a long period of time in a field of dramatic subcellular alterations. The centriole itself is apparently lost irreversibly, and the meiotic divisions are carried out without the participation of a centriole.

Later, microtubular fibers are seen invading the nucleus while others extend laterally into the cytoplasm (PLATES 6; 9E). The **basal nuclear lamina** attains a lobed appearance, finally dissolves, and may be followed by immunohistology as it is drawn in patches into the central region of the cell. The extranucleoli disappear from the nucleus. Their subsequent fate is unclear.

The microtubular system moves, together with the nucleus, toward the animal pole. The nucleoplasm dissipates into the surrounding cytoplasm and the

Structural Changes in the Oocyte

With the advent of MPF activity the morphological transformation of the oocyte to the egg ensues. Although the disappearance of the germinal vesicle is the most prominent feature, actually the whole cell structure is affected. PLATES 4–8 give an impres-

nuclear volume becomes smaller and smaller. Finally, the chromosomes condense and are collected in the first meiotic metaphase spindle (PLATES 6-8; 9F-I).

Due to the absence of the centriole, which has disappeared during oogenesis, the spindle exhibits an uncommon appearance. A normal mitotic spindle, as it forms under the influence of the centriole pair, develops microtubular asters at both spindle poles. These asters are absent in the **maturation spindle** (Fig. 4.2) (PLATE 9I).

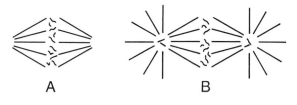

Fig. 4.2. A meiotic (**A**) and a mitotic (**B**) spindle

The unusual structure of the meiotic spindle may aid in polar body formation. Spindle asters in somatic cells are thought to have the function of placing the metaphase chromosomes into a central position within the cell by pushing them away from the cell cortex. They are also thought to define the plane of cell division in the cortex. With fully extended spindle asters it would be difficult to achieve the extremely asymmetric cell division by which the tiny polar body is generated.

The nuclear events of maturation are completed by the first meiotic division and the formation of the first polar body. The second meiotic division is initiated and arrested in the metaphase stage. Haploidization of the maternal genome will be completed after fertilization, when the second polar body is extruded (PLATE 9J,K; 10).

Polar body formation represents an extreme case of unequal cell division. A set of chromosomes is ejected from the oocyte together with a negligible amount of cytoplasm. The biological meaning of this event is obvious. As discussed before, the transcriptional machinery of the oocyte has to work with maximal efficiency to meet the requirements of the steady-state RNA turnover in the huge volume of cytoplasm. It is therefore plausible that the 4C amount of DNA template is maintained in the oocyte until shortly before fertilization to ensure a high rate of transcription. The late haploidization by polar body formation allows the production of large eggs.

The germinal vesicle breakdown is accompanied by a thorough reorganization of the cytoplasm. The subnuclear yolk-free zone expands toward the center of the oocyte (PLATES 5-7). Along its lateral edges, some of the central, large yolk platelets move upwards and are later collected in the spindle region. The packing of yolk becomes loose in the central region, while a tight packing appears lateral to the nuclear area. A zone of "**central yolk-poor cytoplasm**" begins to form. The radii which have been interpreted as yolk-free channels rich in cytoskeletal structures are first distorted before they disappear. Numerous small **yolk-free patches** eventually form within the animal hemisphere (PLATES 8; 10). Immunohistological studies revealed that the nuclear proteins become dispersed in the cytoplasm predominantly of the animal hemisphere.

The cortical region is also affected by the turbulences of maturation. The pigment granules are assembled into denser patches, apparently in some spatial relation to the radii. For some period of time, the pigment layer seems to be drawn slightly into the interior. Later, as the radii disappear, the pigment returns to its original position. This movement does not only affect the animal region but embraces the whole oocyte circumference. The cortical granules are reported to behave in a similar way. The cortex in the vicinity of the metaphase spindle becomes thinner and the pigment granules are displaced. This process generates the white **maturation spot** which provides a clear external sign of successful oocyte maturation (PLATES 7; 8).

As the inner structure of the cell is maintained by the architecture of the cytoskeleton, it is not surprising that this system is significantly affected when the cell structure is remodeled during maturation.

Vimentin is redistributed. The elaborate system of cytokeratin in the vegetal cortex breaks down and disappears. It will reappear after fertilization.

In the cortical region some ultrastructural changes with relevance to future development occur. The junctions between the oocytes and the follicle cells are broken and the microvilli are somewhat retracted. This leads to a considerable decrease in the oocyte surface area. Most remarkable is the development of a cortical endoplasmic reticulum which resembles the sarcoplasmic reticulum of muscle cells in structure. It forms junctional contacts with the plasma membrane and encircles the cortical granules. The system is thought to play an important role in the fertilization process.

In vivo, maturing oocytes are released from the follicle into the peritoneal cavity from where they are transported via the oviduct to the outside pond water. The ion transport systems of the egg plasma membrane have to adapt to the sudden change in the ionic environment. Such adaptations have been reported.

In passing through the oviduct the vitelline layer of the oocyte is altered by the modification and addition of components. The fibrillar mat acquires a smoother appearance in the scanning electron microscope, and the perforations through which the microvilli had contacted the follicle cells disappear. The cell becomes enveloped in a triple-layered jelly coat, consisting of a highly glycosylated matrix cross-linked by disulfide bonds. This matrix quickly swells in the pond water and the egg is ready for fertilization.

A Master Molecule

It is apparent from the description of oocyte maturation, that it involves numerous aspects of the physiology and structure of the oocyte. A way of viewing this event is, that during maturation the cell shifts from one state to the other. The interphase state of the oocyte is maintained by a delicate and unstable balance of molecular interactions. A trigger at the cell membrane sets second messenger systems in motion which are targeted toward a key molecule of the metabolic balance. Once a trace of activated MPF has appeared, the autocatalytic cycle of MPF activation leads to the irreversible manifestation of oocyte maturation. Numerous processes commence by which the intracellular conditions are fundamentally affected until metabolic balance is reestablished in the mitotic state.

The competence of the oocyte to respond to progesterone induction is established during oogenesis. Maturation can therefore be induced only in fully developed oocytes. Oocytes of earlier stages do not respond at all or only aberrantly to progesterone or to the injection of MPF.

The importance of the studies on oocyte maturation may well go beyond their primary goal, which is the understanding of mitosis. Oocyte maturation may quite unexpectedly become a paradigm for a different topic of research namely embryonic induction. The analogy of these two processes is apparent in several aspects.

On their developmental pathway the embryonic cells pass through unstable states during which they are susceptible to specific external signals and competent to respond to them by switching into a different developmental routine. Once this process is initiated, it becomes self-sustaining and independent of the signal.

One may envisage that, in analogy to maturation, the signals are relayed via second messengers to key molecules, whose activity becomes enhanced by autocatalytic cycles and which initiate a cascade of structural and metabolic alterations. When these alterations include multiple changes in gene activity, the developmental program becomes fundamentally reorganized. To dectect and characterize such master molecules in the developing system is the topic of much active research.

References

Reviews

BLOW, J. (1989). Mitosis comes apart. *Trends Gen.* **5**, 166-167.

DUNPHY, W. G. & NEWPORT, J. W. (1988). Unraveling of mitotic control mechanisms. *Cell* **55**, 925-928.

ECKBERG, W. R. (1988). Intracellular signal transduction and amplification mechanisms in the regulation of oocyte maturation. *Biol. Bull.* **174**, 95-108.

HAUSEN, P., WANG, Y. H., DREYER, C. & STICK, R. (1985). Distribution of nuclear proteins during maturation of the *Xenopus* oocyte. *J. Embryol. Exp. Morphol. Suppl.* **89**, 17-34.

KISHIMOTO, T. (1988). Regulation of metaphase by a maturation-promoting factor. *Dev. Growth Differ.* **30**, 105-115.

MALLER, J. L. (1985). Oocyte maturation in amphibians. In *Developmental Biology*, vol.1 (ed. L. W. Browder), pp. 289-311. New York: Plenum Press.

MALLER, J. L. (1985). Regulation of amphibian oocyte maturation. *Cell Differ.* **16**, 211-221.

MASUI, Y. & CLARKE, H. J. (1979). Oocyte maturation. *Int. Rev. Cytol.* **57**, 185-281.

MASUI, Y. & SHIBUYA, E. K. (1987). Development of cytoplasmic activities that control chromosome cycles during maturation of amphibian oocytes. In *Molecular Regulation of Nuclear Events in Mitosis and Meiosis* (ed. R. A. Schlegel, M. S. Halek & P. N. Rao), pp. 1-42. New York: Academic Press.

SMITH, L. D. (1989). The induction of oocyte maturation: transmembrane signalling events and regulation of the cell cycle. *Development* **107**, 685-699.

STICK, R. (1987). Dynamics of the nuclear lamina during mitosis and meiosis. In *Molecular Regulation of Nuclear Events in Mitosis and Meiosis* (ed. R. A. Schlegel, M. S. Halleck & P. N. Rao), pp. 43-66. New York: Academic Press.

WASSERMAN, W. J., PENNA, M. J. & HOULE, J. G. (1986). The regulation of *Xenopus laevis* oocyte maturation. In *Gametogenesis and the Early Embryo*, 44th Symposium of the Society for Developmental Biology (ed. J. G. Gall), pp. 111-130. New York: Alan R. Liss, Inc.

Original Communications

BRACHET, J., HANOCQ, F. & VAN GANSEN. (1970). A cytochemical and ultrastructural analysis of in vitro maturation in amphibian oocytes. *Dev. Biol.* **21**, 157-195.

CAMPANELLA, C., ANDREUCCETTI, P., TADDEI, C. & TALEVI, R. (1984). The modifications of cortical endoplasmic reticulum during in vitro maturation of *Xenopus laevis* oocytes and its involvement in cortical granule exocytosis. *J. Exp. Zool.* **229**, 283-293.

CHARBONNEAU, M. & GREY, R. D. (1984). The onset of activation responsiveness during maturation coincides with the formation of the cortical endoplasmic reticulum. *Dev. Biol.* **102**, 90-97.

HEBARD, C. N. & HEROLD, R. C. (1967). The ultrastructure of the cortical cytoplasm in the unfertilized egg and first cleavage zygote of *Xenopus laevis*. *Exp. Cell Res.* **46**, 553-570.

HUCHON, D., CROZET, N., CANTENOT, N. & OZON, R. (1981). Germinal vesicle breakdown in the oocyte of *Xenopus laevis*: description of a transient microtubular structure. *Reprod. Nutr. Dev.* **21**, 135-148.

LARABELL, C. A. & CHANDLER, D. E. (1989). The coelomic envelope of *Xenopus laevis* eggs: a quick-freeze, deep-etch analysis. *Dev. Biol.* **131**, 126-135.

Chapter 5
Fertilization

During mating, the sperm cells are released into the pond water. They respond to the altered ionic conditions with flagellar movement, which drives them through the jelly coat of the egg. The contact with the jelly material is essential, as it confers to the sperm the capacity to fertilize the egg. This "sperm capacitation" reaction is species-specific and thus provides an interspecies barrier preventing cross-fertilization.

The introduction of the sperm into the egg has several consequences. Its interaction with the egg membrane leads to the egg activation reaction, which is actually the trigger to further development. Furthermore, the sperm endows the egg with a new centriole. As mentioned earlier, this organelle was lost from the egg during oogenesis. Finally, diploidy is restored in the egg by including the paternal genome. We will treat these effects of the sperm on the reacting egg separately in the following.

Restoration of Diploidy

This sperm function, which geneticists would regard as the most important, has the least influence on early embryogenesis. Eggs, fertilized by sperm which was heavily X-irradiated to destroy the paternal genome, develop quite normally, until later on the tadpoles develop the rather unspecific haploid syndrome from which they eventually die.

Egg Activation

This change in the egg constitution, which is triggered by the contact of sperm with the egg membrane, resembles the egg maturation process in several aspects. The reaction is initiated at the plasma membrane, secondary messenger systems are involved, an autocatalytic reaction propagates the response, and many aspects of the physiology of the cell are affected.

Successful fertilization is only achieved when the sperm penetrates the egg surface of the animal hemisphere. Once this has occurred, it is of vital importance for successful development that the entry of further sperm cells is blocked. *Xenopus* has evolved three barriers to fulfill this requirement.

A rapid depolarization of the egg membrane, the "fertilization potential", is induced by the first sperm to arrive at the plasma membrane, and establishes a quick block to polyspermy. This block lasts only a few minutes, but this time is sufficient to erect further barriers against additional sperm cells: The egg surface irreversibly loses adhesiveness for sperm, and the egg integument is altered in such a way as to hinder further sperm cells from approaching the egg.

The decisive event at the membrane that actually triggers the activation reaction is not well understood. Originally, it was assumed that sperm delivers a trace of calcium underneath the plasma membrane. This view was supported by the observation that sperm entry may be mimicked by pricking the egg with a fine needle. Activation is initiated provided that calcium ions are present in the surrounding medium. Likewise, activation may be triggered with calcium ionophores. When intracellular free calcium is artificially lowered by injecting a calcium buffer into the egg, activation is suppressed.

More recent findings suggest that an increased occurrence of free intracellular calcium is a result of a still earlier interaction of a membrane receptor with some sperm constituent, which activates the phosphoinosite second messenger pathway via a G protein. Intracellular free calcium is then released from a store coupled to the membrane reaction system. These assumptions are based on experiments in which a receptor for a neurotransmitter was artificially inserted into the egg membrane. The binding of the ligand to the receptor mimicked sperm-egg interaction and egg activation occurred.

A focus of free calcium at the sperm entry site is the origin of an autocatalytically propagating Ca^{2+} driven wave of Ca^{2+} release, which sweeps over the egg cortex and reaches the opposite pole of the egg within 5−6 min. It is proposed that the subcortical endoplasmic reticulum, which was erected during

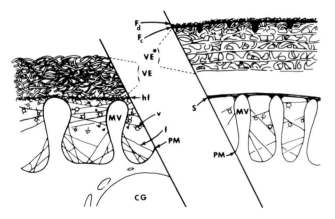

Fig. 5.1. Diagram of the extracellular matrix of the *Xenopus* egg before and after fertilization. The unfertilized egg (*left*) with a cortical granule (*CG*) beneath the plasma membrane (*PM*) and microvilli (*MV*) extending into the perivitelline space. Filaments (*f*) connect MV to each other, to the plasma membrane, and to vesicles (*v*) seen in this region. The vitelline envelope (*VE*) lies on the tips of the microvilli and is attached to them by a layer of horizontal filaments (*hf*) seen at the innermost portion of the VE. After fertilization (*right*), the S layer (*S*) encircles the egg lying on the tips of the microvilli. The VE has elevated and has been chemically and structurally altered (*VE**); the F layer (F_d and F_c) has been deposited on the outer surface of the altered VE. (Larabell and Chandler 1988)

egg maturation, is involved in the sequestration and the release of the Ca^{2+} ions. The progression of this wave front is linked to a wave of a transient contraction of the cortex (PLATE 10). As the "activation wave" passes, the cortical granules discharge their contents into the **perivitelline space** by exocytosis. The vitelline membrane becomes lifted a few microns from the egg surface, and the egg now floats freely in the perivitelline fluid (PLATE 10). Due to the higher density of the vegetal yolk mass, the egg rotates in its envelope until the animal-vegetal axis has become adjusted to gravity, with the animal pole pointing upwards. This orientation ensures an undisturbed development in the next phase, in which the egg plasm gains a higher fluidity. The stratification of the egg cytoplasm is in this way stabilized by gravity. Preventing the egg artificially from rotation often leads to developmental anomalies.

The discharge of the content of the cortical granules into the perivitelline space is required to establish the final block against polyspermy. Granule constituents penetrate the vitelline membrane and react with components of the overlying jelly coat to add a further stable layer to the vitelline membrane. The membrane increases in rigidity; it is now called the "**fertilization membrane**" (Fig. 5.1). The membrane now forms a tight barrier to further sperm cells. It moreover protects the embryo from hazards from the environment, and acts as a corset-like support for the egg.

The rise of free calcium at egg activation is followed by fundamental changes in the cytoplasmic constitution of the egg. Protein synthesis increases twofold. The metaphase arrest is unlocked and the cytoplasm adopts an interphase state in which both the cytostatic factor and the maturation promoting factor lose activity. Again, protein kinase systems in concert with ionic calcium seem to be involved. In preparation for the second meiotic cytokinesis the animal cortex contracts, lifting the pigment border above the equator. This contraction relaxes later. The meiotic division is completed by the formation of the second polar body (PLATES 9J,K; 10). Paternal and maternal chromosomes decondense, and are enclosed by newly formed nuclear envelopes to form the **female** and **male pronuclei**. DNA replication is initiated in the pronuclei. The cortex at the sperm entry site contracts locally, and pigment granules accumulate there at high density, thus marking the **sperm entry point** with a dark spot (PLATE 11).

The Function of the Centriole

The altered conditions in the cytoplasm allow polymerization of tubulin into large microtubular systems. The sperm-derived centriole acts as the nucleation center from which the microtubular **sperm aster** is organized. The aster enlarges gradually and finally extends throughout the whole animal hemisphere (PLATE 11). When the growing aster rays contact the egg cortex, an increase in cortical rigidity causes a change in the outer appearance of the egg surface. The "postfertilization wave" is seen to propagate over the animal hemisphere within 15−20 min.

The microtubular system seems to provide both the

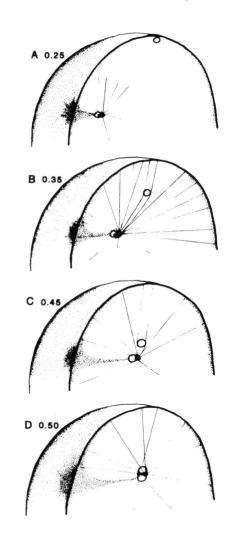

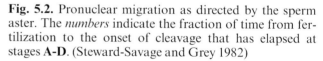

Fig. 5.2. Pronuclear migration as directed by the sperm aster. The *numbers* indicate the fraction of time from fertilization to the onset of cleavage that has elapsed at stages **A-D**. (Steward-Savage and Grey 1982)

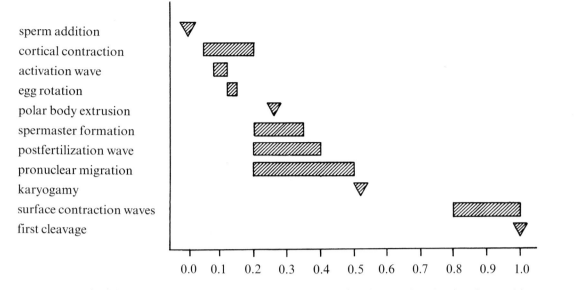

sperm addition
cortical contraction
activation wave
egg rotation
polar body extrusion
spermaster formation
postfertilization wave
pronuclear migration
karyogamy
surface contraction waves
first cleavage

0.0 0.1 0.2 0.3 0.4 0.5 0.6 0.7 0.8 0.9 1.0

Fig. 5.3. Postfertilization events in the *Xenopus* egg on a relative time scale. The time interval between *sperm addition (0.0)* and *first cleavage (1.0)* is 75-90 min depending on the clutch of eggs.

References

Reviews

CHARBONNEAU, M. & GRANDIN, N. (1989). The egg of *Xenopus*: a model system for studying cell activation. *Cell Differ. Dev.* **28**, 71-94.
ELINSON, R. P. (1980). The amphibian egg cortex in fertilization and early development. In *The Cell Surface: Mediator of Developmental Processes* (ed. S. Subtelny & N. K. Wessels), pp. 217-234. New York: Academic Press.
LOHKA, M. J. & MALLER, J. L. (1987). Regulation of nuclear formation and breakdown in cell-free extracts of amphibian eggs. In *Molecular Regulation of Nuclear Events in Mitosis and Meiosis* (ed. R. A. Schlegel, M. S. Halleck, & P. N. Rao), pp. 67-109. New York, London: Academic Press.
LONGO, F. J. (1988). Reorganization of the egg surface at fertilization. *Int. Rev. Cytol.* **113**, 233-268.
SARDET, C. & CHANG, P. (1987). The egg cortex: from maturation through fertilization. *Cell Differ. Dev.* **21**, 1-19.
VACQUIER, V. D. (1981). Dynamic changes of the egg cortex. *Dev. Biol.* **84**, 1-26.

Original Communications

LARABELL, C. A. & CHANDLER, D. E. (1988). The extracellular matrix of *Xenopus laevis* eggs: a quick-freeze, deep-etch analysis of its modification at fertilization. *J. Cell Biol.* **107**, 731-741.
STEWART-SAVAGE, J. & GREY, R. D. (1982). The temporal and spatial relationships between cortical contraction, sperm trail formation, and pronuclear migration in fertilized *Xenopus* eggs. *Roux's Arch. Dev. Biol.* **191**, 241-245.

mobile force and the guidance directing the migration of the two pronuclei toward the center of the animal hemisphere (Fig. 5.2). It appears that the nuclei drag some cortical cytoplasm behind them, so that pigment granules move into the egg interior. The pigmented **sperm trail** marks the pathway of the male pronucleus. The two pronuclei eventually meet near the center of the animal half of the egg (PLATE 12).

The two pronuclei have to move across the large expanse of the animal cytoplasm to meet. The movement must be guided with a high degree of precision, especially since sperm entry may occur anywhere on the animal surface such that the geometrical conditions at the outset of the movement are highly variable between different eggs. The final position of the zygotic nucleus within the eggs is very consistent within a given clutch.

When the two pronuclei fuse, cyclin is resynthesized and MPF activity rises again in preparation for the first cleavage division. A further contraction of the cortex is recorded. A summary and the time scale of the postfertilization events are reproduced in Fig. 5.3.

The analysis of the mitotic and the interphase cytoplasmic states has recently been much stimulated by technical advances. Cytoplasmic extracts may now be prepared from activated eggs, which reproduce many of the effects of egg activation on isolated cellular organelles. These include the formation of chromatin from added DNA, the construction of a nuclear envelope around this chromatin, uptake of nuclear proteins into these artificial nuclei, DNA replication, and the polymerization of tubulin into an aster-like arrangement upon addition of centrosomes. Cyclin mRNAs are translated in the extracts and the accumulation of cyclin protein causes the extracts to shift into a mitotic condition. When nuclei are then added, their envelopes dissolve, DNA synthesis is blocked, the chromosomes condense, and centrosomes induce spindle-like microtubular structures. Thus, these extracts provide a means to study the molecular basis of some of the processes which produce the morphological alterations within egg cells after fertilization, though it is doubtful whether their spatial coordination, as it is revealed by the plates, could ever be explained with this approach.

Chapter 6
Cleavage

During cleavage, development acquires a new quality: a multicellular entity, the blastula, emerges which exhibits a simple but characteristic structure. Initially, this process depends largely on the intracellular organization that has developed during oogenesis and egg maturation. Later on, intercellular cooperation will gradually take over until it becomes the driving force of the developmental progression.

The Cleavage Divisions

In a normal somatic cell, mitotic division is linked to growth: the cell produces its constituents to a level that is sufficient for two daughter cells, and then divides. This is not the case in the developing embryo. As mentioned above, a large store of cellular constituents has accumulated during oogenesis, and there is no need for the egg to rely solely upon its own synthetic machinery. Transcription for example, is not required before the midblastula stage, and development can therefore proceed in the presence of transcription inhibitors. Released from the constraints of the requirement for growth, the cell oscillates rapidly between the interphase and the mitotic state with a cycle length of about 30 min. In contrast to egg maturation and activation, these transitions are not dependent on external triggers; the signals are generated internally.

The pacemaker for the cycles is apparently an oscillatory system driven by the activation and inactivation of MPF. The oscillating system appears to be spread throughout the cytoplasm and works in perfect synchrony in the different regions of the egg, causing the individual cleavage divisions to occur simultaneously within the whole embryo. The egg regions exhibit a high degree of autonomy; no interactions are required to maintain their synchrony. When the newly formed blastomeres are dissociated and separated from each other, they still retain the synchronous rhythm of division. As cleavage progresses the rhythm of the cell cycle within the individual embryonic regions runs somewhat out of phase, such that the cell divisions move over the egg in a wave-like fashion.

When the egg or a blastomere prepares for division, a contraction of the cortex leads to a rounding up of the cell. Later, when the contraction relaxes it falls back into its more flattened ellipsoid shape. This feature is coupled to the cell cycle and may be conveniently used to monitor the characteristics of the oscillating system.

When an egg is divided by ligature into a nucleated fragment which is able to cleave, and a nonnucleated, nondividing fragment, both parts exhibit synchronous cycles of contraction and relaxation. Thus, neither the presence of a nucleus nor the complex events of mitosis are essential for the oscillator's performance. Similarly, when DNA replication is inhibited or tubulin polymerization is suppressed, the oscillator is still active. On the other hand, it is interrupted when protein synthesis is inhibited. This latter result probably reflects the dependence of the MPF function on cyclin synthesis. Using such experiments, events of the cell cycle may be classified into those which are subordinate to the oscillatory system, and those on which the system depends.

The cell cycle of somatic cells is commonly divided into four phases: the G_1 period, the S period of DNA replication, the G_2 period, and the mitotic M phase. The rapid cell cycles during cleavage show no G_1 and G_2 periods, and the S period lasts only 15–20 min. The high rate of DNA synthesis is accomplished by an atypical mode of replication. Strand separation and nucleotide polymerization appear as separate events and long stretches of single-stranded DNA are generated as replication intermediates. The large pool of replicating enzymes and chromatin constituents synthesized during oogenesis ensures that these do not become rate limiting.

Signs of the first cytokinesis are recognizable in the egg about 90 min after fertilization when the first cell cycle has already advanced to the anaphase stage. A pigmented line appears at the animal pole, which deepens to form the **cleavage furrow**. The furrow gradually extends vegetally until it encompasses the whole egg.

The site of the origin of the cleavage furrow at the animal pole is not predetermined within the cortex, but is a result of its interaction with the internal cytoplasm. This can be demonstrated by turning the egg upside down, such that the vegetal pole points upwards. During the phase of cytoplasmic fluidity, the cytoplasm will be reoriented by gravity, and the animal cytoplasm becomes apposed to the vegetal cortex. Cleavage may now initiate in the originally vegetal cortex, and in the best cases further development proceeds as normal.

Information on the position and direction of the cleavage furrow is probably derived from an interaction between the cortex and the cytasters which develop under the influence of the centrioles during mitotic prophase. It might well be that the position of the sperm-derived centriole during the phase of karyogamy is in some way related to the movement of the male pronucleus along the sperm trail. This would explain how the sperm entry site exerts its influence on the position of the first cleavage furrow. In a high percentage of cases the egg divides such that the first cleavage furrow passes through or near the sperm entry site. However, exceptions to this rule are common and have no influence on further development.

PLATE 13 depicts an egg at telophase of the first cleavage division. The animal cortex has contracted and some of the pigment is drawn inwards. Apparently, the future **cleavage plane** is already layed out in the cytoplasm of the animal hemisphere. Cortical material, marked by traces of pigment, is drawn into this plane.

The further events of the first cleavage relate to the forthcoming patterning of the early embryo. In the animal half the cleavage furrow sinks deep into the egg penetrating about one third of its diameter (PLATES 14; 15). At the lower tip of the furrow a small cavity forms, initially still in contact with the outer medium. This cavity represents the **blastocoel anlage**. The formation of this structure seems to be determined by a predisposition of the animal cyto-

plasm. No such modification of the furrow tip is seen in the vegetal region. The position of the future blastocoel is this way linked to the animal-vegetal polarity of the embryo.

The membrane and the underlying cortex of the furrow region contain material derived from the peripheral region of the egg which has been dragged into the interior. The lining of the furrow with pigment granules is a conspicuous manifestation of this movement. Newly formed membrane advances from the site below the presumptive blastocoel, probably by insertion of preformed intracellular vesicles (Fig. 6.1).

The second cleavage furrow forms perpendicular to the first one. The cavities that appear at the new furrow tips fuse with the one formed during the first cleavage, thus enlarging the blastocoel anlage.

PLATES 14 and 15 emphasize how clearly the animal and vegetal fractions of the cytoplasm are now segregated within the egg. The separation of the egg into an animal and a vegetal domain has its origin in the animal-vegetal polarity of the oocyte. It becomes more strongly expressed during maturation and is further enhanced by the cytoplasmic movements during the first and second cleavage.

The third cleavage furrow starts from the prospective blastocoel wall. It advances horizontally and separates the two domains of the egg (PLATE 16). This division is asymmetric such that the embryo now harbors cells of different size, the large **vegetal blastomeres** and the smaller **animal blastomeres**. Although the further divisions are also somewhat asymmetric, this third cleavage division provides the basis for the large difference in size between the animal and vegetal cells of the later blastula, a feature which contributes much to the ultimate pattern of the embryo.

By the time of the third cleavage the blastocoel has expanded considerably. It is sealed off from the outside medium by close junctions which form between the apical regions of contacting cells.

In the vegetal cortical region of the dividing egg small patches of yolk-free cytoplasm appear, which increase in size by fusion, until at stage 4 they form

large yolk-free islands (PLATES 13-16). As this material is later found in the emerging primary germ cells, it has been speculated to play a role in the determination of these cells. The cytoplasmic structure is named **germ plasm** to indicate this supposition. Careful ultrastructural analysis has revealed that this germ plasm relates to the vegetal fragments

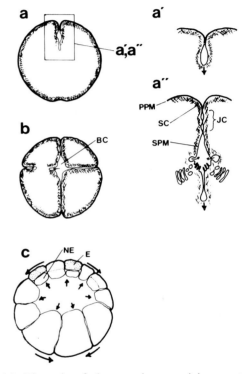

Fig. 6.1. The role of cleavage in organizing anatomical features important to gastrulation. Cleavage occurs partly by furrow formation (**a**,**a′**) and partly by addition of new membrane to the furrow walls by vesicle fusion with the wall (**a″**). A junctional complex (*JC*) forms near the apical edges of the blastomeres and separates the forming blastocoel (*BC*) from the exterior (**a″**,**b**). Tangential cleavages form a superficial epithelial (*E*) and a deep nonepithelial (*NE*) cell population (**c**). The *short arrows* indicate blastocoel expansion, the *long arrows* show expansion of the animal cap and shrinkage of the vegetal region. The apical cell surfaces are derived from the original or primary plasma membrane (*PPM*, *heavy lines*), whereas the deep surfaces of both superficial and deep cells are nascent or secondary plasma membranes (*SPM*, *light lines*). *SC*, subcortical cytoplasm. (Keller 1986)

of the former mitochondrial aggregate, which was a prominent structure in the oogonia and the early oocytes. Its reappearance is another example of how, in spite of the many changes that the cell has undergone since the oogonial stages, traces of structural continuity are being preserved.

A further feature of the cleavage divisions may be recognized in some regions of the sections. At every cell division some material from the cortical region is being transported to the interior along the newly formed membranes. A thin line of pigment granules bordering the inner cell membranes is often the result of this **cortical ingression**. During the later cleavage stages, the germ plasm is also shifted upwards into the interior of the vegetal half as a result of this cortical ingression.

As cleavage proceeds, the cells become progressively smaller, and a number of additional supracellular features arise. The blastocoel is inflated until it comprises about one-eighth of the volume of the embryo. Osmotic forces are thought to be involved in this process. The pumping of Na^+ ions into this cavity followed by passive water influx is one possibility. The osmotic properties of some kind of mucous material, seen in PLATES 17 and 18 as a coarse precipitate, may also contribute to the swelling of the cavity. The blastocoel provides the spatial requirements for the complex cell movements to occur later during gastrulation.

Paratangential cleavage divisions beginning at the 64–128 cell stage generate two new cell types, the cells of the outer epithelial layer and the inner cells. The cells of the outer layer of the blastula become connected by true apical junctional complexes exhibiting tight and intermediate junctions. The embryo is now able to create and maintain an inner ionic milieu, which differs in composition from the surrounding water. From the eight-cell stage onwards, cell coupling via gap junctions is established.

Cleavage thus leads to four easily defined cell types: the animal and the vegetal group of cells, each of which comprises an inner and outer cell population. It will become obvious from the later analysis that the pregastrula pattern may be more subtle than this. Figure 6.1 summarizes the important anatomical features of the cleavage period.

Studies on the cleavage processes have stimulated some discussion on the role of the genome in morphogenetic processes. In the view of common concepts development is driven by the continuous dialogue between the genome and its environment. The individual genes are integrated into a network of communicative interactions within the developing embryo. Changes in the cytoplasmic and extracellular surroundings stimulate new activities of the genomic system, which in turn introduce further changes in the cellular constitution. In this way the developmental progression is sustained.

During cleavage this mutually reflexive dialogue is suspended. Though a low level of transcription is maintained in the cleavage nuclei, there is no evidence that this is strictly required. Cleavage proceeds unimpaired in the presence of inhibitors of transcription up to the late blastula stage. This observation demonstrates the enormous morphogenetic capacity of the activated egg cytoplasm. In the absence of gene activity cells of different sizes and functions arise according to an ordered schedule and cooperate in forming the well-defined morphological entity of the blastula.

It is quite conceivable that this cytoplasmic property of the egg is only an overt example of a more general feature. Cells receiving an external inductive stimulus may well undergo extensive structural and functional changes before the genome reacts to the altered condition. Such considerations tend to ascribe a more responding role to the genome instead of seeing it as the dominant element which controls development.

The Midblastula Transition

Cleavage continues up to the 12th division without apparent changes. The cell cycle length is kept at about 30 min. The recruitment of mRNA for translation that began at oocyte maturation is continued, reaching a level eight times higher than that of the stage VI oocyte. There is apparently not much selectivity in this recruitment; the pattern of polypeptides synthesized remains quite similar. After 12 divisions the store of silent maternal mRNAs runs low, and most of the mRNA is now associated with polysomes. Apart from the movements associated with mitosis the cells are not motile.

At about the 12th cell cycle, 6–7 h after fertilization, the cell cycles lengthen and the synchrony of the divisions breaks down. The rate of transcription per nucleus increases tenfold in the case of the high molecular weight RNA and some 100-fold for the low molecular weight RNA. Some types of maternal mRNAs are selectively recruited for translation. The cells begin to send out lobopodia and filipodia and the whole cell cortex becomes motile. These changes do not occur abruptly, but the time of their appearance is sufficiently short to define these events as a landmark during development, called the midblastula transition (MBT).

The timing of the MBT poses an interesting problem. As described earlier, the cleavage cycles are driven by an oscillating system, the action of which does not depend on the presence of nuclei or on the execution of the whole set of mitotic events. The question to be asked is whether this timing device, which is already operating in the system, is also used to determine the onset of the MBT, i.e., whether the cell cycles are counted.

Evidence is accumulating which indicates that the latter is not the case. The timing of the MBT may be manipulated by methods which do not affect the cell cycle oscillator. In haploid embryos the MBT is delayed by one cell cycle. Removal of three-quarters of the cytoplasm from diploid zygotes by ligature shortens the time which ensues between fertilization and MBT by two cycles. Thus, in contrast to the cell cycle oscillator, the timing of the MBT is influenced by the nucleus. In particular, it is sensitive to the DNA/cytoplasm ratio at the outset of cleavage. MBT is triggered during cleavage when this ratio exceeds a certain value.

A simple titration model may explain the situation.

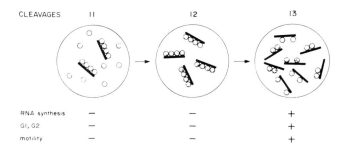

CLEAVAGES	11	12	13
RNA synthesis	−	−	+
G1, G2	−	−	+
motility	−	−	+

Fig. 6.2. The titration model for the midblastula transition. At cleavage 11 excess suppressor molecules (*circles*) are present in the cytoplasm and saturate the DNA template (*bars*). At cleavage 12 the DNA level has doubled and stoichiometric titration is achieved. Subsequent cleavage leads to lack of saturation of the DNA template and activation of transcription. (Newport and Kirschner 1982 b)

The increasing amount of DNA leads to the depletion of some maternal cytoplasmic factor (Fig. 6.2). Once a certain minimal threshold is passed, the MBT is initiated. The exponential mode of DNA accumulation adds to the sharpness of the response. The proposed depletion could be the result of the factor binding directly to DNA, or of its being sequestered into some structure, which relates to the amount of DNA, such as chromatin, nuclear envelope, or nucleoplasm.

Some evidence suggests that the target of the event triggering MBT is the system that controls the cell cycle and that the effects observed at MBT are a consequence of the lengthening of the cell cycle. Inhibition of protein synthesis by cycloheximide blocks the formation of cyclin and thereby the appearance of active MPF after the completion of one further round of DNA replication. The blastomeres are arrested in G_2. Under these conditions, which mimic a prolonged cell cycle, transcription and cell motility can be prematurely initiated.

The concept emerges that at MBT the blastomeres are relieved from the rapid succession of cell cycles driven by the oscillator. With the lengthening of the cell cycle and the advent of a G_1 and G_2 period, conditions are established to allow for orderly gene activation and regulation. Prior to MBT the transcriptional machinery might have been impaired by the unusual mode of rapid DNA replication. Gene activation at MBT seems to be partially selective. Some novel RNA species have been detected, but the bulk of transcription corresponds to genes which had previously been active in the oocyte.

Spare time between cell divisions might also permit the cytoskeleton to become involved in cell motility. The onset of translation of certain species of maternal mRNA, e.g., fibronectin, histone I, or lamin II, adds to the impression that the physiological conditions within the blastomeres are fundamentally affected. Some of the individual processes initiated at the MBT seem to be quite independent of each other. For instance, the change in cell motility and the selective translation of the above mentioned mRNAs occur perfectly well in embryos inhibited in transcription by antimetabolites.

It has been repeatedly pointed out how the construction of the oocyte is directed toward the formation of the early embryonic spatial pattern. The control of the MBT demonstrates that also the timing of the embryonic events is under the influence of properties of the oocyte which are established during oogenesis.

The new conditions set the stage for the next phase of development; cell movements begin to occur in the embryo, aided by the presence of newly formed extracellular material. New cell contacts are established organizing a system of intercellular communication. As a response new territories arise within the embryo which become stabilized by establishing their specific pattern of gene activity.

References

Reviews

BENBOW, R. M. (1985). Activation of DNA synthesis during early embryogenesis. In *Biology of Fertilization* (ed. C. B. Metz & A. D. Monroy), pp. 246-299. New York: Academic Press.

COOKE, J. & SMITH, J. C. (1990). Measurement of developmental time by cells of early embryos. *Cell* **60**, 891-894.

DIXON, K. E. (1981). The origin of primordial germ cells in the amphibia. *Neth. J. Zool.* **31**, 5-37.

EDDY, E. M. (1975). Germ plasm and the differentiation of the germ cell line. *Int. Rev. Cytol.* **43**, 229-280.

ETKIN, L. D. (1988). Regulation of the midblastula transition in amphibians. In *Developmental Biology*, vol. 5 (ed. L. W. Browder), pp. 209-225. New York: Plenum Press.

KELLER, R. E. (1986). The cellular basis of amphibian gastrulation In *Developmental Biology,* vol. 2 (ed. L. W. Browder) pp. 241-327. New York: Plenum Press.

KIRSCHNER, M., NEWPORT, J. & GERHART, J. (1985). The timing of early developmental events in *Xenopus. Trends Genet.* **1**, 41-47.

LASKEY, R. A. (1985). Chromosome replication in early development of *Xenopus laevis. J. Embryol. Exp. Morphol.* **89**, 285-296.

NIEUWKOOP, P. D. & SUTUSURYA, L. A. (1979). *Primordial Germ Cells in the Chordates Embryogenesis and Phylogenesis.* Cambridge: Cambridge University Press.

Original Communications

BALLARD, W. W. (1955). Cortical ingression during cleavage of amphibian eggs. *J. Exp. Zool.* **129**, 77-98.

BLUEMINK, J. G. & DE LAAT, S. W. (1973). New membrane formation during cytokinesis in normal and cytochalasin B-treated eggs of *Xenopus laevis. J. Cell Biol.* **59**, 89-108.

BYERS, T. J. & ARMSTRONG, P. B. (1986). Membrane protein redistribution during *Xenopus* first cleavage. *J. Cell Biol.* **102**, 2176-2184.

GAUDETTE, M. F. & BENBOW, R. M. (1986). Replication forks are underrepresented in chromosomal DNA of *Xenopus laevis* embryos. *Proc. Natl. Acad. Sci. USA* **83**, 5953-5957.

KALT, M. R. (1971). The relationship between cleavage and blastocoel formation in *Xenopus laevis*. I. Light microscopic observations. *J. Embryol. Exp. Morphol.* **26**, 37-49.

KALT, M. R. (1971). The relationship between cleavage and blastocoel formation in *Xenopus laevis*. II. Electron microscopic observations. *J. Embryol. Exp. Morphol.* **26**, 51-66.

NAKAKURA, N., MIURA, T., YAMANA, K., ITO, A. & SHIOKAWA, K. (1987). Synthesis of heterogeneous mRNA-like RNA and low-molecular-weight RNA before the midblastula transition in embryos of *Xenopus laevis*. *Dev. Biol.* **123**, 421-429.

NEWPORT, J. & KIRSCHNER, M. (1982a). A major developmental transition in early *Xenopus* embryos: I. Characterization and timing of cellular changes at the midblastula transition. *Cell* **30**, 675-686.

NEWPORT, J. & KIRSCHNER, M. (1982b). A major developmental transition in early *Xenopus* embryos: II. Control of the onset of transcription. *Cell* **30**, 687-696.

SANDERS, E. J. & SINGAL, P. K. (1975). Furrow formation in *Xenopus* embryos. Involvement of the Golgi body as revealed by ultrastructural localization of thiamine pyrophosphatase activity. *Exp. Cell Res.* **93**, 219-224.

SINGAL, P. K. & SANDERS, E. J. (1974). An ultrastructural study of the first cleavage of *Xenopus* embryos. *J. Ultrastruct. Res.* **47**, 433-451.

SINGAL, P. K. & SANDERS, E. J. (1974). Cytomembranes in first cleavage *Xenopus* embryos. Interrelations between Golgi bodies, endoplasmic reticulum and lipid droplets. *Cell Tissue Res.* **154**, 189-209.

WARNER, A. (1989). The role of gap junctions in amphibian development. *J. Embryol. Exp. Morphol. Suppl.* **89**, 365-380.

Chapter 7
Gastrulation

A decisive and dramatic event during early development is the process of gastrulation. It comprises a set of complicated morphogenetic movements from which the embryo emerges as a bilateral individual, in which the three distinct germ layers, ectoderm, mesoderm and endoderm are clearly layed out. A new system of body axes is erected under the influence of both the original animal-vegetal polarity and a cue for bilateral symmetry, which has been present in the embryo since fertilization. Anterior and posterior as well as dorsal and ventral regions of the embryo become clearly marked. Gastrulation establishes the basic vertebrate body plan in the embryo.

The basic methods to investigate gastrulation were established by the early experimental embryologists and are still commonly in use though adapted to modern fashion and technology. A prerequisite for any experimental study is the detailed morphological analysis of the gastrula at different stages. Further techniques include the construction of fate maps by following dye-marked regions of the pregastrula through gastrulation and the assessment of their morphogenetic potential by transplanting and explanting specific regions of the early gastrula. These experiments also allow conclusions on the autonomy or mutual dependency of the individual processes.

In spite of considerable efforts the details of gastrulation are still not understood, but a rough outline can be given. A proper appreciation of the well-ordered choreography of the intertwined movements of the individual embryonic territories calls for much spatial imagination, especially, since the different processes are interlocked and occur simultaneously. One way to facilitate the description is to divide the pregastrula into regions which exhibit definable traits of morphogenetic movements and to treat these separately. In addition, the influences imposed upon the system by the animal-vegetal polarity may be distinguished from those derived from the cue of bilateral symmetry mentioned above. In this way the complexity of the system may be reduced. Once the pattern of the movements and their

mechanics are understood, the system may be open to a further reduction and analysis at the cellular level, in order to understand the behavior of cell groups from the properties of their individual members.

Pregastrula Movements

Pregastrula movements start in the blastula stage, when the **blastocoel roof** is still a multilayered sheet three to four cells in depth with the superficial cells connected by tight junctions (PLATE 17). The cells of the blastocoel roof are all derived from the animal hemisphere of the egg. They collectively perform the movement of epiboly, by which the vegetal hemisphere becomes partially covered with animal material. While retaining their epithelial junctions, the cells of the outer layer stretch and become thinner, thus increasing the animal surface. During this process none of the inner cells become inserted into the outer epithelium. Instead, these cells interdigitate by radial intercalation to form the single-celled inner layer of the blastocoel roof. Due to this cell rearrangement the expansion of the deep layer is more efficient than that of the superficial layer, and the two layers slide past each other. As a result of the whole process, material from the animal half, in particular from the inner layer, is transported vegetally and a multilayered ring of originally animal cells forms in the subequatorial region. To compensate for this movement the superficial vegetal cells constrict their apices, thus keeping the surface of

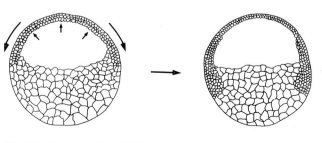

Fig. 7.1. Pregastrula epiboly

the embryo smooth. The inner yolky vegetal cells are shifted upwards to a certain extent (Fig. 7.1).

Gastrulation

At the onset of gastrulation the embryo can be subdivided into different regions on the basis of their characteristic types of cell behavior. The assembly of the individual regions in the embryo is illustrated in Fig. 7.2a and each region is depicted separately in Fig. 7.2b-f. The **animal cap** (AC, Fig. 7.2b) comprises the upper half of the blastocoel roof. The lower half of the animal material is called the **marginal zone** (MZ). It is further subdivided into the upper **noninvoluting marginal zone** (NIMZ; Fig. 7.2c) and the multilayered ring of subequatorial cells, the **involuting marginal zone** (IMZ). This zone contains three layers, the **deep zone** (DZ; Fig. 7.2d) adjacent to the vegetal yolk mass, a **subepithelial layer** (Fig. 7.2e) and the superficial, **epithelial layer** (Fig. 7.2f). The **vegetal yolk mass** is not further subdivided. These regions will be treated separately in the following description of gastrulation. It should be emphasized that the definition of the regions is somewhat arbitrary as clear borders cannot easily be defined and the different zones tend to merge at the boundaries.

We begin the explanation with a fictitious, radially symmetric embryo, in which gastrulation is exclusively governed by the original animal-vegetal axis and all movements occur in accordance with this symmetry. For didactic reasons we shall ignore all other influences for the time being.

The animal cap continues epiboly and will eventually cover about half of the embryo (Fig. 7.2b-b'). The NIMZ initially shows an activity similar to the epiboly of the AC, but as it extends vegetally a new form of movement occurs. The cells interdigitate circumferentially along the parallels of latitude, a behavior called "convergence". This results in a constriction of the circumference of the NIMZ ring of cells as it is shifted vegetally. At the same time the whole NIMZ is stretched by "extension" in the ani-

mal-vegetal direction, thereby giving the mantle a cup-shaped appearance (Fig. 7.2c-c'). The AC and the NIMZ together ultimately cover the whole surface of the embryo.

The involuting marginal zone exhibits the most complex morphogenetic movements. The deep zone begins to move already before the onset of gastru-

lation is externally visible, and these cells probably come to occupy their deep position by an internal involution, a process called "cryptic gastrulation". During gastrulation these cells display a characteristic "spreading" behavior (Fig. 7.2d-d'). They migrate as a coherent sheet over the blastocoel roof, which serves as the adhesive substratum for their

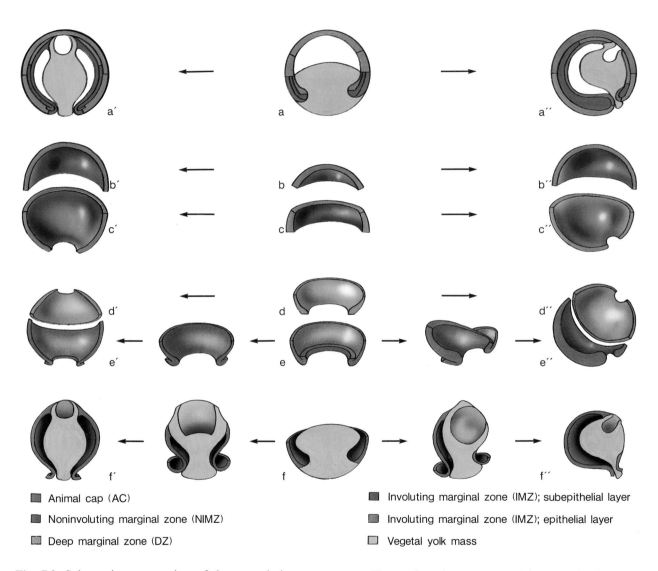

Animal cap (AC)

Noninvoluting marginal zone (NIMZ)

Deep marginal zone (DZ)

Involuting marginal zone (IMZ); subepithelial layer

Involuting marginal zone (IMZ); epithelial layer

Vegetal yolk mass

Fig. 7.2. Schematic presentation of the gastrulation movements. For explanation, see text. Diagrams in the top row represent sagittal sections through the embryo at the pregastrula (**a**) and the late gastrula stage (**a',a''**). Diagrams **a'-f'** illustrate gastrulation movements as they would occur in a fictional, radially symmetrical embryo, whereas **a''-f''** show the conditions in a normal, bilaterally symmetrical embryo.

migration. The deep cells will eventually cover the upper part of the blastocoel roof.

In addition to the deep cells, the IMZ consists of the outer epithelial layer and the multilayered subepithelial sheet of cells. This latter cell group shows a unique behavior (Fig. 7.2e-e'). It moves upwards toward the blastocoel roof in the wake of the deep zone, but in order to do so the sheet of cells has to roll over an inner blastopore lip, a process called "involution". As the successive levels of this sheet involute, they show increasingly stronger convergence by circumferential cell intercalation. This movement occurs after the cells have passed the lip of involution at a time when the gastrulation is already well under way. It leads to an increasing constriction of the ring of converging cells. Cells would pile up in this ring of convergence if this movement were not counterbalanced by a second vector of movement called "extension", in which the cells move along the parallels of longitude. Radial and circumferential intercalation aid this movement. In fact, all movements occur simultaneously and the whole maneuver is therefore named "convergent extension" (Fig. 7.3). The movement is sustained by the inherent mechanical properties of the cell sheet as no substratum for migration is required. The tensile forces which are generated by this process are thought to be counterbalanced by the mechanical rigidity of the vegetal yolk mass which is being driven inwards and "overrolled" by the lip. Convergent extension of the subepithelial IMZ seems to be the principal driving force in the vegetal movement of the blastopore and its constriction.

The superficial layer of the IMZ is translocated to the inside of the embryo by the gastrulation movement (Fig. 7.2f-f'). In our fictitious embryo a ring of cells at the vegetal border of the superficial marginal zone, about 50° off the equator, will start gastrulation by constricting their apices. This constriction concentrates the pigment of the apical cortex to form a dark ring within the vegetal hemisphere. It represents the outline of the **blastopore**. These **bottle cells** extend into the interior and apparently make contact with the DZ cells. It is likely that bottle cells

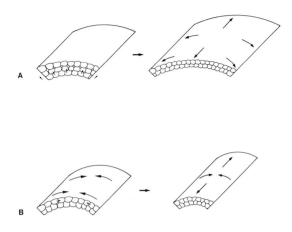

Fig. 7.3. Epiboly (**A**) and convergent extension (**B**)

facilitate the involution of the subepithelial IMZ in the initial stage.

In concert with the deep zone and the bottle cells the epithelial layer of the IMZ moves into the embryo by involuting round the outer **blastopore lip**, and ultimately encloses the whole yolk mass. At the expense of the blastocoel a space is inflated between the yolk mass and the involuted superficial layer. In this way the **archenteron** forms. With the progression of gastrulation the ring of involution constricts and moves downwards, driven by the forces of convergent extension of the subepithelial IMZ material. When the borderline between NIMZ and IMZ reaches the outer lip, the involution ceases, the blastopore is closed (Fig. 7.2f-f'). In Fig. 7.2a' the different territories have been reassembled into the final construct.

This symmetrical model describes many features of the gastrulation process. As a general rule, cells move as fairly coherent groups, and there is no excessive intermingling between the territories. This lack of extensive cell mixing has allowed the construction of fate maps of the pregastrula.

At the end of gastrulation the ectoderm, which is derived from the outer and inner layer of animal cells, covers the entire embryonic body. The archenteron is bounded by the endoderm, which is derived from the suprablastoporal superficial IMZ, and by

the epithelial border of the vegetal yolk mass, which originates exclusively from the vegetal half. The bottle cells have respread and add to the archenteron wall. The layer between ectoderm and the endodermal epithelium forms the mesoderm which is also derived from animal material, but exclusively from the inner cells.

The processes just described would create an embryo which is symmetrical with reference to the animal-vegetal axis. Only little has to be added to adapt the model to reality and to make the system diverge from radial symmetry to express the required bilateral symmetrical features.

One source of asymmetry arises from the differential timing of the gastrulation movements around the egg circumference. At the onset of gastrulation, the pigmented band of the bottle cell apices first appears on one side. This band represents the first obvious mark of the future dorsal side of the embryo. A plane of bilateral symmetry passing through this mark may be constructed. The formation of the bottle cells and the gastrulation movements, which begin on the dorsal side, then propagate laterally until they reach the opposite ventral side about 2 h later. When the gastrulation movements cease, the pattern generated by these movements remains much more advanced on the dorsal side than on the ventral side.

The other trait which leads to the emergence of bilateral symmetry is an asymmetry in the character of the convergent extension movement of the ring of subepithelial IMZ material. Convergent extension is a directed movement. Material is transported from the lateral and ventral regions of the subepithelial IMZ toward the dorsal midline and, by extension, the thickened and elongated rod of dorsal axial mesoderm is formed (Fig. 7.2e-e''). Dorsal convergence begins midway through gastrulation, first on the dorsal midline and then spreads laterally. Similarly, the convergence of the NIMZ is a directed movement, which generates a shift of lateral cells to the dorsal midline, where they engage in the formation of hindbrain and trunk neural tube. Recent observations have indicated that convergent extension of the NIMZ is acquired through an inductive interaction with the adjacent IMZ at the preinvolution stage. Therefore, the NIMZ represents a region of autonomous behavior from only the midgastrula stage onwards, after this induction has occurred.

The differential timing of the movements and the directed convergence have a number of consequences for the ultimate structure of the gastrula. The mantle of spreading mesoderm comes to occupy an oblique position (Fig. 7.2e″). More posteriorly the massive rod of the axial mesoderm occupies the middorsal region. Due to the retarded involution and dorsal convergence little of the mesoderm showing convergent extension remains ventral to the blastopore. The archenteron forms preferentially at the dorsal side; its dorsal and lateral walls are represented by the endoderm derived from the superficial IMZ and respread bottle cells. Only a slight indication of the archenteron is seen on the ventral side. The vegetal yolk mass is tilted. Part of it forms the archenteron floor. Due to the earlier and more vigorous involution at the dorsal side, the blastopore is shifted ventrally (Fig. 7.2 a″).

The plane of bilateral symmetry, which we were able to define at the onset of gastrulation, persists throughout the gastrulation process and defines the plane of symmetry of the future animal. At the end of gastrulation, the movements have generated a definite dorsal and ventral side marked by the position of the axial mesoderm and the ventral yolk mass. The closed blastopore represents the posterior end of the anterior-posterior axis.

The position of the individual parts of the body which may be described within this anterior-posterior and dorsoventral axial system bears little relation to their original position in the primitive axial system. For example, as a consequence of the involution, material originally positioned vegetally below the equator comes to lie close to the original animal material in the anteriormost region, whereas other parts of the vegetal material lie in the ventral posterior region. Similarly material from other body regions is shifted toward the dorsal side. To

clarify the situation it would seem practical and legitimate to state: A new axial system is erected during gastrulation and the primitive axial system is discarded while the plane of symmetry is preserved. We have retained, however, the commonly used terminology: the side on which the dorsal axial system is formed coincides with the side on which the onset of gastrulation is seen. This side is termed the "dorsal" side also of the pregastrula embryo, the opposite side is called the "ventral" side. The term animal-vegetal axis is abandoned for the postgastrula stages.

The harmony of the various gastrulation movements suggests that they are all interdependent, generating a whole which directs and regulates the behavior of the individual regions. However, a large body of investigations indicates that the individual regions exhibit an appreciable degree of autonomy and that the embryo at the pregastrula stage represents a mosaic of territories, each endowed with different formative tendencies which they express in due time. The autonomous behavior is, however, expressed in an environment, which poses constraints on the individual cell groups and this interaction modulates the outcome of the autonomous traits.

These conclusions are derived from experiments in which the behavior of embryonic regions is studied in isolated explants. Their behavior in the context of a new environment can also be investigated in heterotopic or heterochronic transplants. Finally, ablation experiments give information on how the behavior of a given region influences its surroundings.

Animal caps, isolated at the onset of gastrulation, will round up, expand, and generate folds. They differentiate into "atypical epidermis". It is not clear whether this behavior can be viewed as epiboly which is aberrant due to the lack of the tension normally imposed onto this region by the inflated blastocoel. In situ the outer animal cap cells stretch and flatten, and the cells of the inner layer interdigitate, which results in the spreading of the whole. Which of these two processes, if either of them, provides

the driving force for the epibolic movement cannot be decided.

The spreading of the deep zone may be observed when blastocoel roofs together with the adhering migrating cells are explanted from early gastrulae of appropriate stages. Time-lapse films demonstrate the migration of these cells in a broad front. The questions being investigated concern the substratum for the adhesion and migration of the cells and the cues which guide the direction of their movements. At the onset of gastrulation, the blastocoel roof is already covered by a network of extracellular matrix. One prominent component of this matrix is fibronectin, which is synthesized in the late blastula and preferentially deposited on the blastocoel roof. The participation of this component in the adhesion and migration of the cells has been inferred from experiments using inhibitors of the interaction of the cells with fibronectin. It is possible that the stretching of the blastocoel roof by epiboly confers a directionality to the matrix network which is utilized to guide the migrating deep zone cells.

The behavior of the bottle cells provides another example of a process with a regionally specific autonomy, which is modulated by surrounding influences. In situ, the bottle cells exhibit a unilateral apical constriction and an elongation of the cell body extending into the vegetal cell mass. After moving to the inside of the embryo they respread to deepen the archenteron. In isolation these cells constrict and spread out again at the same time as they would have done in situ. There is, however, a morphological difference. In isolation their apical surfaces become rotund instead of stretched laterally as is the case in situ. Thus, two fundamental properties of the bottle cells, apical constriction and respreading, follow an autonomous program. Its realization in situ leads to alterations of the cell shape due to the mechanical influences of the surrounding tissue.

The autonomy of the gastrula territories can also be observed by explanting a strip of embryonic tissue from an early gastrula extending from the blastopore up to the animal pole. In the course of further development the deep cells leave the explant and form a ball of mesenchymal cells. The adjacent regions, which correspond to IMZ and NIMZ, become separated by a distinct border. They show narrowing and elongation by convergent extension. The region of the animal cap forms a vesicle of atypical epidermis. Much of this behavior reflects the in situ situation.

From the midgastrula stages on, the individual regions begin to express differentiation tendencies in relation to their future fate. The animal cap derivatives on the surface of the embryo will develop into epidermis and the anterior nervous system. The trunk neural tube derives mostly from the NIMZ. The population of spreading cells from the deep zone is the precursor of the head mesoderm and much of the lateral and ventral part of the mesodermal structures. The subepithelial IMZ showing convergent extension will form the axial system of notochord and somites. The dorsal and lateral lining of the archenteron will differentiate into endoderm, and the vegetal yolk mass will end up in the gut where it will be digested and used as the primary food supply.

Many of the features outlined in this description may be recognized in PLATES 18-25. However, it is not easy to discern all the details. Endodermal and mesodermal cells are still very similar in character and not easily distinguished morphologically, nor are the individual territories separated clearly enough to define the borders unequivocally.

The Organizer

In 1924, Hilde Proschold in Spemann's laboratory performed an experiment which caused decades of excitement and discussion. The dorsal suprablastopore lip of a newt gastrula was transplanted into the corresponding ventral site of another embryo. The implant performed normal gastrulation movements and caused the formation of a whole set of dorsal and lateral structures in addition to those of the host. A double embryo developed with the ventrolateral regions joined. In addition, the experiment demonstrated that it was not only the transplant that gave rise to the secondary embryonic structure, but that host tissue participated in the formation of the "secondary embryo" to a considerable degree. Because the experimental manipulation was in fact a common assay for induction processes and a whole embryo was "induced" by this transplantation, the event was termed the "primary induction" and the suprablastoporal region was called the "organizer". Both terms were misleading. The first one denied that there could be other inductive events prior to gastrulation, a notion which curtailed the interest in earlier events. The second term unconsciously introduced a vitalistic concept to the field, evoking the supposition of an entity, which was sculpturing the embryo from the virgin cell mass of the blastula "like an artist creating a sculpture or a painting" (Spemann). Views have changed since then, but the enigmatic nature of the original observation has remained.

The experiment has been repeated many times and the phenomenon was systematically investigated also in the *Xenopus* embryo. In the preceding description the early gastrula was viewed as a mosaic of cell groups which exhibit a high degree of autonomy with respect to their morphogenetic tendencies. The organizer transplantation demonstrates another feature of the embryo: the capacity to regulate the fate of individual regions with their cells being able to adapt to a new context. Under the influence of the transplanted organizer the marginal zone, which was fated to become ventral mesoderm, now forms the dorsal mesoderm of the secondary embryo. The secondary dorsal mesoderm in its turn induces dorsal ectodermal structures at ectopic sites.

The orderly positioning of the new mesodermal structures suggests that the mesodermal mantle behaves according to the rules of a regulative morphogenetic field which is organized by some kind of a global positional information system. The transplanted organizer region seemingly acts as the new center of such a field. Some observations agree with the formalism of this theory, others pose a challange.

The capacity of the assumed field to regulate seems to be limited. Complete excision of the organizer results in the complete suppression of the formation of axial mesoderm. A radially symmetrical embryo forms and the whole mesoderm expresses the lateral and ventral features of the spreading cell population. Partial excision of the organizer results in the formation of defective axial structures. When an implanted organizer is brought into close proximity to the host organizer, the preexisting host organizer does not establish dominance over the implant as would be expected from a regulating field; initially both organizers are acting independently. Later, the two developing axes fuse in quite a harmonious manner. The field of the mesodermal mantle is not isomorphic. Rotation of the organizer region by 90° leads to an abortive excrescence, regulation does not occur. This result indicates that the inherent polarity of the mesodermal mantle is retained after implantation.

It is difficult to subsume all these observations within a comprehensive model and different hypotheses may be put forward. Among other ideas, it is conceivable that the decisive function of the organizer is to act as a center of directed convergent extension. As described above, convergent extension in the subepithelial IMZ causes a polarized dislocation of prospective mesodermal cells from lateral and ventral positions toward the organizer region. An implanted second organizer may likewise attract cells from the surrounding region and integrate them into the emerging rod of mesodermal cells. Furthermore, it is conceivable that, once started, this process is self-enhancing and propagates into the adjacent tissue. The suprablastoporal region may merely provide the initiating cue for this cell behavior. In the course of the gastrulation movements numerous changes occur with respect to the patterns of cell shape, cell contacts, or regional cell density. Anyone of these parameters or a combination of them may provide the spatial cues to establish a prepattern of mesoderm organization, which is stabilized and reinforced when different groups of cells respond to the information entailed in their position by establishing specific patterns of gene activity. Inductive influences of the mesoderm then transfer spatial information to the adjacent germ layers.

References

Reviews

GERHART, J. & KELLER, R. (1986). Region-specific cell activities in amphibian gastrulation. *Annu. Rev. Cell Biol.* **2**, 201-229.

HOLTFRETER, J. F. (1988). A new look on Spemanns' organizer. In *Developmental Biology*, vol. 5 (ed. L. W. Browder), pp. 127-150. New York: Plenum Press.

KELLER, R. E. (1986). The cellular basis of amphibian gastrulation. In *Developmental Biology*, vol. 2 (ed. L. W. Browder), pp. 241-327. New York: Plenum Press.

KELLER, R. & HARDIN, J. (1987). Cell behaviour during active cell rearrangement: evidence and speculations. *J. Cell Sci. Suppl.* **8**, 369-393.

NAKAMURA, O. & TOIVONEN, S. (eds.) (1978). Organizer - A Milestone of a Half-Century from Spemann. Amsterdam: Elsevier/North-Holland Biomedical Press.

WITKOWSKI, J. (1985). The hunting of the organizer: an episode in biochemical embryology. *TIBS* **1**, 379-381.

GERHART, J., DANILCHIK, M., DONIACH, T., ROBERTS, S., ROWNING, B. & STEWART, R. (1989). Cortical rotation of the *Xenopus* egg: consequences for the anteroposterior pattern of embryonic dorsal development. *Development Suppl.* **107**, 37-51.

Original Communications

COOKE, J. (1972). Properties of the primary organization field in the embryo of *Xenopus laevis*. I. Autonomy of cell behaviour at the site of initial organizer formation. *J. Embryol. Exp. Morphol.* **28**, 13-26.

COOKE, J. (1972). Properties of the primary organization field in the embryo of *Xenopus laevis*. II. Positional information for axial organization in embryos with two head organizers. *J. Embryol. Exp. Morphol.* **28**, 27-46.

COOKE, J. (1972). Properties of the primary organization field in the embryo of *Xenopus laevis*. III. Retention of polarity in cell groups excised from the region of the early organizer. *J. Embryol. Exp. Morphol.* **28**, 47-56.

COOKE, J. (1973). Properties of the primary organization field in the embryo of *Xenopus laevis*. IV. Pattern formation and regulation following early inhibition of mitoses. *J. Embryol. Exp. Morphol.* **30**, 49-62.

COOKE, J. (1973). Properties of the primary organization field in the embryo of *Xenopus laevis*. V. Regulation after removal of the head organizer, in normal early gastrulae and in those already possessing a second implanted organizer. *J. Embryol. Exp. Morphol.* **30**, 283-300.

COOKE, J. (1989). Mesoderm-inducing factors and Spemann's organiser phenomenon in amphibian development. *Development* **107**, 229-241.

KELLER, R. E. (1975). Vital dye mapping of the gastrula and neurula of *Xenopus laevis*. I. Prospective areas and morphogenetic movements of the superficial layer. *Dev. Biol.* **42**, 222-241.

KELLER, R. E. (1976). Vital dye mapping of the gastrula and neurula of *Xenopus laevis*. II. Prospective areas and morphogenetic movements of the deep layer. *Dev. Biol.* **51**, 118-137.

KELLER, R. & TIBBETS, P. (1989). Mediolateral cell intercalation in the dorsal axial mesoderm of *Xenopus laevis*. *Dev. Biol.* **131**, 539-549.

NAKATZUJI, N. (1975). Studies on the gastrulation of amphibian embryos: cell movement during gastrulation in *Xenopus laevis* embryos. *Roux's Arch. Dev. Biol.* **178**, 1-14.

NIEUWKOOP, P. D. & FLORSCHUETZ, P. A. (1950). Quelques caractères spéciaux de la gastrulation et de la neurulation de l'oef de *Xenopus laevis* Daud. et de quelques autres anoures. I. Etude descriptive. *Arch. Biol.* **61**, 113-150.

Chapter 8

The Emergence of the Pregastrula Pattern

In Chapter 6 the development of the blastula morphology was viewed as a process largely determined by the conditions established in the egg during oogenesis. The description of gastrulation has then revealed that an elaborate pattern of autonomous territories, which are characterized by their inherent morphogenetic potential, is concealed within the overt morphology of the late blastula. The two most important features of this pattern are a cue of bilateral symmetry, which breaks the original radial symmetry around the animal-vegetal axis, and secondly the specific properties of the prospective mesoderm cells of the marginal zone, which provide the major driving forces for gastrulation. Other features of the blastula are important as well, but their morphogenetic role in the gastrulation process is less pronounced.

The question as to how this pattern of territories arises in the pregastrula phase is a topic of much active research. For a long time these investigations were retarded by methodical limitations, a situation that is changing at present. Some of the methods used are still those of the classical period of embryology: pieces of embryonic tissue are explanted or transplanted and the differentiation tendencies of these pieces are then used to define their state of commitment for a specific developmental pathway. Classically, morphological and histological analyses are used to score for such differentiation tendencies. The influence of certain blastula territories on others may be assayed by combining different explanted pieces in vitro. By varying the timing of the experiment the emergence of characteristic regional differentiation potencies during cleavage may be investigated.

The problem with this kind of analysis is that histological differentiation is a relatively late event. One has to rely on the assumption that the conditions for autonomous cellular differentiation are already set at the time of the initial experimental manipulation and that they are not established afterwards by secondary interactions within the explant. It is therefore desirable to obtain information on the region-specific differentiations of an isolate as soon as possible after its removal from the embryo in order to reduce such secondary effects.

Molecular techniques are now being applied to find probes which can be used reliably as early markers of region-specific cell differentiation. Most of the markers obtained are either antibodies directed against tissue-specific components such as actin for somitic muscles, neurofilaments or N-CAM for neural cells, and cytokeratins for epidermal cells, or cDNA probes generated from the mRNA of such molecules. Compared to histological criteria these probes allow a somewhat earlier identification of the onset of cell differentiation. However, it seems extremely difficult to obtain region-specific molecular markers for the different territories of the pregastrula. It is possible that the molecular differences are only minor at these stages: the differential cell behavior at gastrula may be brought about not so much by the formation of new molecules, but more by modifications and spatial reorganization of preexisting components.

The Formation of the Prospective Mesoderm

The analysis of gastrulation has revealed that the main driving force of this process resides in the prospective mesoderm of the involuting marginal zone. Due to the eminent role of this cell population in organizing the basic body plan, much effort has been devoted to elucidate its emergence during the pregastrula phase. The result is a quite elaborate analysis of the first inductive event in the embryonic development.

The mapping of the pregastrula movements indicates that the prospective mesodermal cells are derived from the animal region. A simple experiment shows, however, that the capacity of the animal material to form mesoderm is not inherited from a predisposition localized in the animal hemisphere of the egg. The third cleavage plane separates the animal and the vegetal compartment of the early embryo. If an embryo is divided along this cleavage plane to yield the animal and the vegetal quartet of blastomeres and the pieces are cultivated separately in a balanced salt solution, the animal piece differentiates into atypical epidermis, the vegetal piece forms an unstructured cell mass, but neither of them develops mesodermal characteristics.

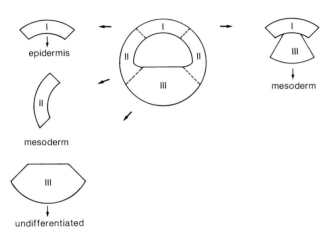

Fig. 8.1. Regions of the blastula used to demonstrate *mesoderm* induction

A similar experiment may be performed at the mid-blastula stage. The embryo is divided into three regions as depicted in Fig. 8.1. Only the marginal region (II) forms mesodermal tissue in isolation. The animal cap region (I) and the vegetal region (III) behave like the corresponding pieces of the eight-cell embryo. If, however, regions I and III are combined and cocultivated, they form an aggregate in which typical mesodermal differentiations occur such as the formation of notochord, muscle, or blood. A closer analysis using labeled animal or vegetal explants reveals that the mesoderm is derived exclusively from the animal material as is also the case in the intact embryo.

These observations provided the basic evidence for the notion that the prospective mesoderm arises from an induction of animal cells by the vegetal region, the animal material being the responsive part and the vegetal material emitting a signal. Additional experiments have shown that animal and vegetal material need to be in contact for about 2 h to elicit a maximal response, and that the animal cap cells are responsive to the signal during the period from early blastula up to the beginning of gastrulation. This time interval comprises the period of competence for this induction.

Although the whole animal cap is responsive to the vegetal signal during the period of competence, the prospective mesoderm of the embryo is confined to a narrow ring at the lower edge of the blastocoel wall, a topological feature which is essential for an ordered progression of gastrulation. The blastocoel seems to serve the important function of insulating the majority of the animal cells from the vegetal influence. Apparently, the vegetal signal can only spread a short distance through the lateral wall of the blastocoel.

Based on these results investigations into the chemical nature of the inducing signal have been carried out. Animal caps excised from late blastulae serve as an assay system. They are supposed to react upon the addition of compounds with signal activity by differentiating mesodermal tissue characteristics. Molecular probes indicative of mesoderm are particularly useful to test for differentiation in these assays.

Although *Xenopus* embryos can be obtained by the thousands, the quantities are not sufficient to allow the characterization of inducing compounds, which may be present in minute amounts as would be expected for such signaling molecules. It was therefore attempted to circumvent this problem by testing readily available heterologous material for mesoderm inducing capacity. A bewildering variety of positive results was obtained with such exotic material as extracts from guinea pig bone marrow or carp swimbladder.

The recent finding that polypeptide growth factors from different sources possess mesoderm-inducing activity explains these earlier observations, when the ubiquitous distribution of these factors and their phylogenetic conservation is taken into account. The importance of the discovery that growth factors or growth factor-related compounds participate in induction lies in the fact that molecules known to act as signals in the adult are also engaged in embryonic cell interactions. The whole body of knowledge of the effects of growth factors on their target cells, which has accumulated in quite diverse areas of research, can now be applied to the induction process. For instance, it may be anticipated that the intracellular transduction pathways of growth factor signals are similar in embryonic and adult cells.

Surprisingly, a variety of growth factors which have diverse effects in different systems are active in mesoderm induction. One group comprises various members of the fibroblast growth factor class (aFGF, bFGF, kFGF, int-2 oncogene product), a second group is the transforming growth factor ß class (TGF-ß1, TGF-ß2, XTC-MIF). None of the factors found to be active in the induction assays has yet been proven to be the natural inducer within the embryo.

As described before, an RNA species termed vg-1 is synthesized during oogenesis and is strictly localized along the vegetalmost cytoplasm of the late oocyte stages. Its nucleotide sequence shows similarity to TGF-ß growth factor mRNA. The translation product of this RNA, which has yet to be identified, is a prominent candidate for the natural inducer, the more so as its localization within the embryo is at a site expected to be the source of the inducing signal.

The concept emerging from these observations is that during cleavage the polar anisotropy in the egg establishes two cell lines, which generate the animal and the vegetal cell population, both endowed with their own specific differentiation tendencies. In the course of development, the vegetal cells emit growth factor-like molecules as signals which are received by the adjacent animal cells. The propagation of these factors through the tissue is limited, such that only a ring of animal cells in the marginal zone is induced. The blastocoel insulates the rest of the animal cap from the vegetal influence. The induced animal cells respond to the signal by diverging from their autonomous progression toward epidermal differentiation and by establishing the capacity to perform their specific function in gastrulation, during which they come to form the mesoderm.

During gastrulation it becomes apparent that the marginal zone is not a homogeneous ring of cells but consists of several populations of cells each exhibiting a specific behavior. The inner material forms the deep zone with the spreading cells and the zone of cells exhibiting the convergent extension behavior. The superficial epithelium of the involuting marginal zone comprises a ring of prospective endodermal cells. In addition, the noninvoluting marginal zone exhibits a distinct behavior. Whether these different cell types are elicited by one single induction event, perhaps by some graded distribution of the signal, or whether secondary interactions within the induced marginal zone are required to elaborate the pattern remains unclear.

In addition to this pattern, different regions around the circumference of the ring of the prospective mesoderm acquire different properties. The emergence of this latter feature is discussed in the context of the second important trait of pregastrula pattern formation, the establishment of bilateral symmetry.

The Origin of Bilateral Symmetry

During gastrulation, the animal-vegetal axis and a plane of bilateral symmetry serve as the reference coordinate system to organize the processes spatially. When gastrulation begins with the apical constriction of the bottle cells at the future dorsal side, the bilateral symmetry of the embryo becomes overtly expressed. Its emergence during the preceding developmental period is referred to as the process of symmetrization. In principle, all that is required to define bilateral symmetry in the embryo is a region of unique property localized away from the animal-vegetal axis. A plane passing through this region and through the animal-vegetal axis would then define the new plane of symmetry (Fig. 8.2). The required singularity would also define the polarity of the new axis.

Assuming that the egg does not contain some hidden internal cue, bilateral symmetry could in principle be established by two quite different mechanisms. An external cue may introduce the required region of unique property. Alternatively, the bilateral character may arise spontaneously by a true symmetry breaking process, i.e., the field, isotropic with respect to the egg's or embryo's circumference, shows some stochastic fluctuations of its properties, which may eventually trigger a self-enhancing process at any location, leading to the manifestation and stabilization of the requested singularity. Experimental evidence shows that, depending on the circumstances, either of the mechanisms can elicit symmetrization in the *Xenopus* egg.

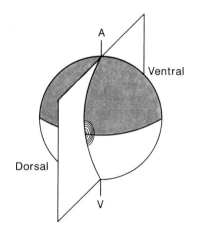

Fig. 8.2. A plane of bilateral symmetry passes through the animal-vegetal axis and a singularity off this axis

Under normal conditions, sperm entry provides an external signal which evokes symmetrization. The sperm entry site in the animal hemisphere of the egg is marked by a dark spot of contracted cortex. Following the fate of this site up to gastrulation reveals that it labels the future ventral side of the embryo. This shows that the plane of symmetry is already defined in the fertilized egg.

By applying sperm to the egg with a micropipette, it can be demonstrated that sperm can enter anywhere in the animal hemisphere. Thus, the future dorsoventral polarity of the embryo can be manipulated by the experimenter proving that the egg does not possess a predetermined plane of symmetry, but that this is introduced at fertilization. A more detailed analysis reveals that the correlation between the sperm entry point and the future plane of symmetry is not very strict, as if the causal connections between the two were not stringent. It seems that the sperm entry canalizes an independent symmetry-evoking mechanism with variable success.

If fertilized eggs are exposed to a pulse of UV light from the vegetal side, or to hydrostatic pressure or low temperature, the process of symmetrization is blocked. Development of the eggs is initiated normally, but gastrulation is severely affected. The embryos assume a radially symmetrical pattern throughout, resulting in postgastrula stages lacking bilateral symmetry and dorsal axial mesoderm; only ventral mesodermal structures are produced. The resulting structure reminds us of the fictitious embryo depicted in Fig. 7.2a'.

If the animal-vegetal axis of an UV-treated egg is tilted to 90° off its normal perpendicular orientation in the field of gravity, the heavy vegetal yolk slides downwards, and the whole cytoplasm rotates within the shell of the egg membrane and cortex. Under these conditions the defects provoked by UV treatment are cured, and normal embryos develop. Moreover, the direction of the cytoplasmic movement is truly predictive of the future dorsal midline of the embryo.

Labeling the peripheral cytoplasm of the egg with a spot pattern of vital dyes makes it possible to monitor the displacement of cytoplasm within the cortex under normal conditions. The experiments reveal that, starting at 30 min postfertilization and lasting up to 75 min postfertilization, a rotation of the cytoplasm relative to the cortex occurs such that the vegetal yolk shifts some 30° toward the sperm entry site. Again, the direction of the movement is predictive of the future plane of symmetry.

A microtubular system is established in the vegetal subcortical region during this period. The individual fascicles are aligned with the direction of the cytoplasmic movement, indicating that the rotation may indeed be accomplished by the microtubules. Presumably, this system is impaired by the treatments which block symmetrization. It appears, therefore, that the directed displacement of cytoplasm relative to the cortex is causally linked to the symmetrization process, which, on the other hand, is influenced by the entry of the sperm from the outside. An indication of the cytoplasmic rotation is the displacement of internal pigment granules versus the unpigmented cortex of the equatorial region of the egg, which is to be seen in PLATES 11 and 12.

Under experimental conditions, bilateral symmetry may arise from a true symmetry-breaking process. When an egg, from which the maturation spindle has been removed, is artificially activated in the absence of sperm, cytoplasmic rotation occurs nonetheless, but this time in a random direction. It is possible to stimulate such eggs to undergo normal development by implanting a nucleus and a centriole. In this case the dorsal midline of the future embryo can be predicted from the direction of the rotation that had occurred before the implantation of the nucleus.

All of these observations and data may be subsumed in the following model: in its subcortical layer the egg possesses a system to polymerize tubulin upon egg activation. The emerging microtubules orient themselves in a common, but random, direction by a kind of self-organization. Possibly, the first nucleation events in the polymerization process are decisive and propagate their direction into the surrounding region. Under the influence of the sperm centriole the sperm aster forms at one side of the animal half. It is quite conceivable that the two microtubular systems interact in such a way that the sperm aster imposes a spatial cue on the subcortical microtubular system. The polymerized microtubules drive the rotation of the cytoplasm within the cortex. This rotation triggers a response which leads to a stable difference in the cytoplasmic conditions between two sides of the egg. This difference anticipates the future dorsal and ventral regions. One can only speculate on the nature of the imme-

diate reaction triggered by the cytoplasmic shift. Surely, new neighborships arise at the cortical-cytoplasmic border which may lead to new molecular interactions, but the decisive events have not been identified as yet.

The Dorsoventral Specification of the Prospective Mesoderm

Using the sperm entry point as a marker, the future dorsal and ventral side of the embryo may be predicted with reasonable certainty. This feature has been exploited to characterize the effects of symmetrization on the pregastrula pattern.

Symmetrization adds a further element of regional mosaicism to the pattern specified by the animal-vegetal polarity. If an eight-cell embryo is divided into two halves along the dorsoventral plane of symmetry, the "right" and the "left" fragments regulate and develop into normal, half-sized embryos. If, however, the future dorsal half is separated from the ventral half, the former differentiates anterodorsal structures and the latter ventral structures only.

These findings connect symmetrization with the process of mesoderm induction. Various experiments indicate that the vegetal cells of the dorsal side have the capacity to induce a cell population programmed for the dorsal mesoderm pathway in the animal region. The vegetal cells of the ventral side induce ventral mesodermal structures. This effect is most easily seen when the animal cap of an early blastula prior to mesoderm induction is rotated by 180°. The dorsal side of the future embryo is determined by the vegetal and not by the animal cells. The experiment may be repeated with isolated dorsal and ventral vegetal blastomeres which are combined with animal caps. The recombinant explants differentiate dorsal and ventral mesodermal features according to the origin of the inducing vegetal cells (Fig. 8.3).

The question arising from these observations is whether the different responses provoked by the

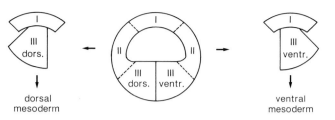

Fig. 8.3. Demonstration of the polarized organization of the vegetal regions inducing *dorsal* and *ventral mesoderm*

dorsal and ventral vegetal cells are due to different "dorsal" and "ventral" signaling factors or whether it is the signal intensity that varies. Experiments with growth factors give an ambiguous answer. XTC-factor induces more dorsal structures at high concentrations and more ventral structures at lower concentrations, indicating that a graded concentration of one factor may be sufficient for the patterning of the mesoderm. On the other hand, bFGF induces only ventral structures, indicating that in this case additional qualities are required for the complete pattern.

The reaction of the animal cap cells to the inducing factors gives further insight into the process of mesodermal pattern formation. Regardless of whether isolated animal caps are exposed to the inducing factor or whether the factor is injected into the blastocoel, the cells respond by a change in behavior. "Dorsalizing" but not "ventralizing" conditions elicit a response in vitro which is reminiscent of the convergent extension movement of the dorsal mesoderm in situ. Animal cap explants elongate and stretch out. A group of animal cells that has been exposed to dorsalizing conditions displays organizer activity when transplanted ventrally into a host gastrula.

The timing of the response of the animal cells to the inductive stimulus depends on their own autonomous program. Regardless of the time of induction, the reaction is always observed when the responding cells are due to undergo gastrulation in situ. In fact, cells induced to form dorsal structures display a response at the early gastrula stage and "ventralized" cells do so at midgastrula, indicating that the timing of the response depends on the fate for which the cells are programmed during induction.

In the intact embryo a dorsoventral difference in the timing of certain pregastrula events anticipates the earlier appearance of the blastopore on the dorsal side. Gap junctions between the blastomeres are first formed at the 32-cell stage with a preference to the dorsal side. Transcription during midblastula transition is initiated more strongly on the dorsal side, and the pregastrula movements are also somewhat stronger on the dorsal side. These effects cannot be due to an enhancement of general metabolic activity on the dorsal side. Experimental acceleration of the development of the ventral side by controlled warming does not result in a reversal of the dorsoventral axis.

Combining these diverse observations, one arrives at the following model of how the breaking of radial symmetry by the rotation of the egg cytoplasm may exert its influence on the prospective mesoderm during gastrulation: The cytoplasmic rotation elicits an anisotropy in the vegetal region, which in the blastula stages leads to an asymmetrical release of mesoderm-inducing factors to which the animal cells react. The signal is either stronger on the future dorsal side, or chemically different. According to their own timing schedule, which depends on their degree of "dorsalization", the induced cells respond with changes in behavior. A center of convergent extension is established on the dorsal side, which spreads its influence far into the lateral and ventral region and recruits cells for the formation of the axial mesoderm on the dorsal side. The remaining ventral mesoderm is derived mainly from spreading deep cells, which do not participate in convergent extension. The decisive influence producing the bilateral symmetry of the gastrulation process is exerted by the suprablastoporal material. It is not known how far other regions of the embryo are independently biased toward bilateral symmetry.

A further fundamental question concerns the relations between the pregastrulation pattern and the future fate of the embryonic regions. Are the prospective mesodermal cells already committed to a specific differentiation pathway such as notochord or muscle by the induction at the pregastrula stage and are the following morphogenetic movements only an expression of this commitment? Or does the commitment of the prospective mesodermal cells initially only program a specific cell behavior? In this case the multiple cell interactions, the changes in cell shape, and cell density patterns, which occur during gastrulation, may be used as an information system to program the position-specific differentiations of the individual cell groups.

References

Reviews

DAWID, I. B., SARGENT, T. D. & ROSA, F. (1990). The role of growth factors in embryonic induction in amphibians. *Curr. Top. Dev. Biol.* **24**, 262–284.

ELINSON, R. P. (1989). Microtubules and specification of the dorsoventral axis in frog embryos. *Bioessays* **11**, 124-127.

ELINSON, R. P. & KAO, K. R. (1989). The location of dorsal information in frog early development. *Dev. Growth Differ.* **31**, 423-430.

GERHART, J. C., VINCENT, J. P., SCHARF, S. R., BLACK, S. D., GIMLICH, R. L. & DANILCHIK, M. (1984). Localization and induction in early development of *Xenopus*. *Philos. Trans. R. Soc. Lond.* [Biol.] **307**, 319-330.

GURDON, J. B. (1987). Embryonic induction - molecular prospects. *Development* **99**, 285-306.

GURDON, J. B., MOHUN, T. J., SHARPE, C. R. & TAYLOR, M. V. (1989). Embryonic induction and muscle gene activation. *Trends Genet.* **5**, 51-56.

KNOECHEL, W. & TIEDEMANN, H. (1989). Embryonic inducers, growth factors, transcription factors and oncogenes. *Cell Differ. Dev.* **26**, 163-171.

NIEUWKOOP, P. D. (1973). The organization center of the amphibian embryo: its origin, spatial organization and morphogenetic action. *Adv. Morphog.* **10**, 1-39.

SMITH, J. C. (1988). Cellular interactions in establishment of regional patterns of cell fate during development. In *Developmental Biology*, vol. 5 (ed. L. W. Browder), pp. 79-120. New York: Plenum Press.

SMITH, J. C. (1989). Mesoderm induction and mesoderm-inducing factors in early amphibian development. *Development* **105**, 665-677.

WAKAHARA, M. (1989). Specification and establishment of dorsal-ventral polarity in eggs and embryos of *Xenopus laevis*. *Dev. Growth Differ.* **31**, 197-207.

WOODLAND, H. R. (1989). Mesoderm formation in *Xenopus. Cell* **59**, 767-770.

YAMANA, K. & KAGEURA, H. (1987). Reexamination of the 'regulative development' of amphibian embryos. *Cell Differ.* **20**, 3-10.

Original Communications

BACHVAROVA, R. & DAVIDSON, E. H. (1966). Nuclear activation at the onset of amphibian gastrulation. *J. Exp. Zool.* **163**, 285-296.

BLACK, S. D. (1989). Experimental reversal of the normal dorsal-ventral timing of blastopore formation does not reverse axis polarity in *Xenopus laevis* embryos. *Dev. Biol.* **134**, 376-381.

NAGAJSKI, D. J., GUTHRIE, S. C., FORD, C. C. & WARNER, A. E. (1989). The correlation between patterns of dye transfer through gap junctions and future developmental fate in *Xenopus*: the consequences of u.v. irradiation and lithium treatment. *Development* **105**, 747-752.

VINCENT, J. P. & GERHART, J. C. (1987). Subcortical rotation in *Xenopus* eggs: an early step in embryonic axis specification. *Dev. Biol.* **123**, 526-539.

Chapter 9

The Shaping of the Body Pattern during the Gastrula and Neurula Stages

Although they overlap in time and are causally interconnected it is appropriate to distinguish, at least formally, those processes in the gastrula which drive and exert the gastrulation movements proper from those which use the novel conditions within the embryo to initiate new traits of development. The most prominent of these latter events are the structural patterning of the mesoderm and the formation of the neural anlage. In general, the development of the mesoderm is the leading process on which others depend through inductive interactions.

The Mesoderm

As described in the previous chapter, the mesodermal mantle of the late gastrula derives from two cell populations, which are already distinct at the onset of gastrulation. One population, the spreading cells, which are localized deep in the marginal zone of the early gastrula, forms the anterodorsal prechordal plate from which the head mesoderm originates. Further, the spreading cells give rise to most of the lateral plate and all of the ventral mesoderm. Prominent differentiations are the heart, the kidneys, and the blood-forming system.

The second population consists of the cells of the subepithelial marginal zone. They display convergent extension and eventually form the compact rod of **axial mesoderm**, which will differentiate into the central notochord and the two portions of flanking paraxial somitogenic material. Whereas the differentiation tendencies of the spreading cell population become obvious only later, the axial mesoderm exhibits overt morphogenesis already during gastrulation.

The Axial Mesoderm

Convergent extension in the dorsal mesoderm continues far into the neurula stages, giving rise to a disproportionate elongation of the dorsal side of the embryo. This results in a stretching and transient bending of the embryo. During this period material is added to the axial mesoderm from a thick "**circumblastoporal collar**" by involution and radial intercalation.

The development of the axial structures has been studied by conventional histology, by scanning electron microscopy, and by filming of explants in which the morphogenetic movements continue unimpaired. Signs of **notochord** formation can already be seen in the blastoporal region right after the first axial mesoderm has involuted. Using the scanning electron microscope a difference between the prospective notochord and the paraxial cells is visible as early as at stage 11^+. The notochordal cells are flatter and more tightly packed and extend lamellar protrusions to contact their neighbors. The paraxial cells are separated by larger intercellular spaces and connected by filiform protrusions. These features indicate that the two populations initially differ in cell contacts and adhesiveness. The boundary between the two structures is vague at first, but becomes more prominent at stage 12 (PLATE 22B). By convergent extension the notochordal anlage is elongated at the expense of width and pushed anteriorly. In fact, the extension of the notochord is greater than that of the adjacent paraxial mesoderm, such that notochordal cells slide past the paraxial cells. At the same time cells are continuously added to the posterior notochordal anlage by radial and circumferential intercalation which leads to a further extension along the dorsal midline.

From stage 13 onwards the notochord becomes surrounded by a network of extracellular material, which will eventually form the notochordal sheath. Typical extracellular matrix components such as laminin, fibronectin, and proteoglycans are found in this sheath. From stage 23 onwards the notochordal cells become highly vacuolated (PLATE 36). Their turgescence adds to the stability of this supportive element of the embryonic axis. The notochord is only a transient embryonic organ but has been implicated in a number of important developmental processes, such as neural induction, the morphogenetic shaping of the neural plate, and the induction of various mesodermal differentiations.

Two longitudinal ridges of **paraxial mesoderm**, also called **somitogenic mesoderm**, are formed on either side of the notochord by convergent extension. They will eventually become segmented into individual somites. This process is preceded by changes in cell morphology and cell arrangement. In the late gastrula stages, the cells begin to elongate and become oriented mediolaterally. These changes in cell shape and cell behavior begin at the anterior end of the paraxial mesoderm and propagate posteriorly in a wave-like fashion. Some of these features are clearly recognizable in PLATES 22B, 23, 28, 30, 33. The difference between the regular cell orientation of the paraxial mesoderm and the random orientation of the cells in the **lateral plate mesoderm** becomes obvious at stage 14 (PLATE 23).

Observing the formation of these axial structures in situ one gets the impression that the well-organized morphogenetic movements depend on the delicate topographical arrangement of the cells within the gastrulating embryo. A particularly impressive experiment indicates that this dependence is not so strict, but that the formative processes are endowed with a high degree of self-organizing capacity.

In this experiment late blastulae, about to initiate gastrulation, are dissociated into single cells in a Ca^{2+}-free medium. After complete scrambling of the cells, they are reaggregated by addition of Ca^{2+}. After a while the aggregates begin to elongate and to form protrusions, they obviously undergo some kind of morphogenesis. Histological analysis reveals, among other structures, stretches of well-formed notochord, which is often accompanied by paraxial mesoderm in a manner which resembles the in vivo situation. Explanted animal caps induced to form mesoderm behave likewise. Thus, axial structures and other elements of the final pattern can even form in the complete absence of a preformed topography. The spatial order in which the individual structural elements are arranged in the aggregates is, however, grossly disturbed. The execution of the gastrulation movements seems to be necessary to achieve the proper order of pattern elements.

The above result is probably not due to a sorting out of predetermined cells. If the cells are kept dispersed, none of them will differentiate muscle- or notochord-specific characteristics. Thus, the cells at the early gastrula stage are not so rigidly determined that they can perform their developmental programs in isolation. Their differentiation to a terminal state depends on the intercellular cooperation within an aggregate. Once they have received their specification in the aggregates, they can be readily cultivated as single cells which will express their specific differentiation tendencies. Such observations support the idea that also in situ the final commitment for a specific differentiation occurs by cell cooperation during gastrulation.

Somitogenesis

Segmentation is a basic feature of the vertebrate body, being overtly expressed in the vertebral column, the structure of the trunk central nervous system, and the arrangement of the trunk musculature. This characteristic pattern originates during the neurula stages when the two ridges of paraxial mesoderm lining the notochord begin to subdivide into the repetitive pattern of the **somites**. A remarkably regular process generates tissue blocks of equal size in a precisely timed sequence, which starts in the anterior region and propagates posteriorly in a wave-like fashion.

Two aspects of the segmentation process shall be treated separately: Firstly, the individual somite is separated from the continuous tissue strand of paraxial mesoderm by a most remarkable set of morphogenetic movements, which requires a detailed morphological analysis to be understood. Secondly, the overall pattern of segments seems to be generated by some general coordinative mechanism. The control of number and size of the somites and their formation in an exactly timed sequence are being investigated. These studies also relate to the problem as to how these processes are linked to the mesoderm formation during gastrulation.

Morphogenesis of a Somite

At the onset of somite formation, the lateral as well as the paraxial mesoderm is double-layered, the two regions being clearly distinguished by cell shape and arrangement. The two cell layers of the presomitic mesoderm are separated by a **myocoelic slit**, the first coelomic cavity found in the embryo. The cells are elongated and radiate from the slit bending toward the dorsal midline. In the vicinity of the notochord the cells lie at right angles to the anterior-posterior axis (PLATES 28; 30; 33).

In the following stage slight changes in the cell rearrangements occur. The dorsalmost cells of the paraxial mesoderm change shape and begin to segregate from the more ventral mass. This dorsal material does not participate in somite formation, it forms the **dermatome** which remains unsegmented in *Xenopus* (PLATES 33; 35; 37; 38) and later forms the dermal layer of the skin.

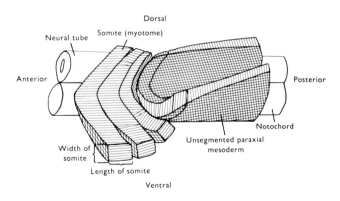

Fig. 9.1. Three-dimensional reconstruction of somite formation in *Xenopus*. The axial and paraxial structures are viewed from a ventrolateral position on the *left-hand side*. Blocks of paraxial mesodermal cells are shown in the process of reorientation that accompanies somite formation. (Hamilton 1969)

Blocks of somitogenic material, measuring about 10 cell diameters in anterior-posterior direction, now undergo a coherent movement which results in their detachment from the rest of the mesodermal ridge and in a 90° rotation of the whole block, such that the cell tips, which were adjacent to the notochord, come to point anteriorly. In this way, the length of the so-formed somite along the anterior-posterior axis is determined by the length of its constituent cells, and the width is determined by the original anterior-posterior extension of the block of cells. Immediately after rotation the newly formed somite becomes enveloped in a sheath of basal lamina. Figure 9.1 shows the whole process as reconstructed from serial sections and PLATES 35 and 37 give examples of somites in rotation. It should be noted that other vertebrates, and even other amphibians, use different strategies to construct their somites, although the starting situation and the result of the maneuver are very similar.

The Somite Pattern

The first somite is formed in the neurula at stage 16-17 in the anterior trunk region (PLATE 29). Then segmentation proceeds in a wave propagating caudally at a speed of one somite per 40 min. The pattern that arises is very regular, the width of the somite in terms of cells per diameter remains constant throughout the trunk region. The length of the somites, determined by the length of the constituent cells, varies somewhat as the body axis stretches, with the cell lengths adjusting to these conditions. The segmentation pattern is strictly in accord with other aspects of the body pattern, the limb buds, for instance, always appear at the level of a given somite.

The formation of a somite does not depend on the prior formation of its anterior neighbor, i.e., the wave passing over the mesoderm is not self-propagating as it is the case for most of the well-known waves in our physical environment. Removal of a piece of presomitic mesoderm, or even slicing the embryo into an anterior and posterior half, does not impair the passage of the wave of segmentation into the posterior piece at the right time. The term "cinematic wave" has been coined for this behavior. The observations indicate that the time sequence of the formation of the segments and the location of the boundaries are already precisely preset in the paraxial mesoderm, the wave front being only the verification of a preformed pattern.

This raises the question when and under which circumstances the prepattern is layed down. The finding that certain conditions, such as a short treatment with nocodazole (an antitubular drug) or a short exposure to high temperature (37.5 °C), will transiently impair the basic patterning mechanism, allows an estimate. After such a pulse treatment, four to six somites are formed as usual, followed by a region of one or two ill-defined or distorted segments after which normal somites appear again. This result indicates that the foundations of the individual segments are laid at least 160 to 240 min before they appear morphologically; segmentation of the anterior mesodermal region dates back to the time, when the paraxial ridge is being formed during gastrulation.

Beginning at midgastrula and extending into the neurula and postneurula stages, axial mesoderm is continuously generated in the blastoporal region. After involution the cells of the circumblastoporal collar first pass through a region where they intercalate radially, then through a second region where the anterior-posterior extension is driven preferentially by circumferential intercalation, which continuously narrows the rod of axial mesoderm. In the paraxial strands the process comes to a halt, when the cells have elongated and become oriented toward the newly formed notochord. At this stage somite formation begins. Figure 9.2 depicts this progression. It seems plausible that the wave of segmentation is only the final expression of a sequential program of cell behavior through which the paraxial mesoderm passes after involution around the inner blastoporal lip.

It is therefore likely that the foundation of the seg-

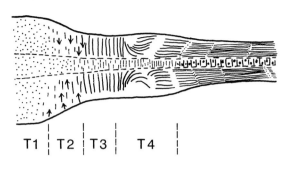

Fig. 9.2. During somite formation each level of the axial mesoderm passes the stages T_1-T_4. At T_1 extension is driven preferentially by radial intercalation, at T_2 by circumferential intercalation, at T_3 cell orientation changes, at T_4 somite formation by rotation commences. (After Cooke and Zeeman 1976)

ment pattern is laid down during the time when the cells are still engaged in convergent extension before they settle in their final position along the axis. Detailed scanning electron microscope analysis of the presomitic mesoderm of the gastrula has revealed that an inkling of segmentation may already be recognized at this stage. The paraxial mesoderm is said to be subdivided into an array of somitomeres.

Later in development the four anteriormost somites are obliterated. This takes place at stage 25, when the ear vesicle forms in this region. Segmentation and somite formation in the outgrowing tail continue far into the tadpole stages. The cellular material is generated by cell division in the terminal zone of the tail. In this zone the segments are determined before they can be morphologically distinguished. The mechanism seems to be similar to that in the gastrula/neurula phase.

Normally, embryos exhibit some variation in size. The body size of an embryo may be experimentally manipulated by removing material from the late blastula. Under all these conditions the number of somites remains constant, their size being adjusted to the quantity of cells available. The system forming the segmentation pattern has the ability to regulate.

The fundamental importance of the process of segmentation, its spatial and temporal precision, and the inherent regulative capacity have challenged investigators to construct models, which might explain the features of the system. Different intuitive and mathematically founded models have been proposed such as a "gradient positional information" system, a "clock wave front" model, and others based on induction. A closer discussion of this topic is beyond the intention of this text. The reader is referred to the literature cited below.

The Beginning of Neurogenesis

The formation of the neural anlage is an easily recognizable external feature of the developing embryo. At stages 11/12 the inner layer of the dorsal ectoderm, extending from the blastoporal region toward the animal pole, begins to thicken and to bulge slightly, which is the first indication of **neural plate** formation. Its delineations sharpen until at stage 15/16 the lateral borders begin to converge to form the neural folds. This process starts from the posterior end and indicates the onset of neural tube formation. The regionalization of the central nervous system becomes externally visible during stages 18/19. Neurulation ends with neural tube closure at stage 20.

Two aspects of this process have received the particular attention of embryologists. Studies on neural induction seek to explain how the dorsal gastrula ectoderm is determined to leave the pathway toward epidermal differentiation and to enter the neurogenic pathway and how the neural plate is regionalized into increasingly diverging structures. The second aspect concerns cell shape changes, the morphogenetic movements, and the "mechanics" of neural tube formation. It may be anticipated that these two aspects of neurulation encompass many common features and overlap to a large extent.

Neural Induction

The formation of the neural anlage in the dorsal ectoderm depends on inductive tissue interactions during gastrulation. If the ectoderm is isolated from mesodermal influences, no neural tissue differentiates. If a piece of isolated ectoderm is combined with a block of gastrula dorsal mesoderm, neural differentiation is observed. Upon implantation of a second organizer an additional neural plate forms at an ectopic site as a result of the inducing influence.

Due to the ease with which the inducing and reacting components can be obtained and because of the complex pattern that results from their interaction, neural induction is a particularly attractive system to study. Unfortunately, *Xenopus* is not as suitable for this work as are other amphibians. Since in *Xenopus* the individual developmental processes occur so rapidly and overlap in time, the limits of temporal resolution become an important source of ambiguity in the experiments. This is one reason why most of our knowledge on amphibian neural induction is derived from observations on urodeles (*Ambystoma*, *Triturus*). The basic model that has emerged from these classical studies probably also applies to *Xenopus*, although details are certainly different. One obvious difference relates to the morphological conditions at the outset of neurogenesis. In urodeles the reacting ectoderm is a unicellular layer, whereas in *Xenopus* it is two cell layers thick. Secondly, a different mode of mesoderm formation may further contribute to the differences between *Xenopus* and the urodeles. Nevertheless, a short outline of the conclusions derived from classical experiments on urodeles may be appropriate in the current context.

The animal cap ectoderm is competent for neural induction during the phase extending from the late blastula up to the midgastrula stage; thus, the competences for mesodermal and neural induction overlap for a significant period of time. This fact initially caused confusing conflicts in this area of research, since an early mesoderm induction, leading

through secondary interactions to neuralization, may easily be misinterpreted.

A first wave of neural induction is generated by the prechordal plate mesoderm as it moves along the dorsal midline of the gastrula, provoking the differentiation of the overlying ectodermal cells into the columnar generative neuroepithelium of the neural plate. In the absence of further influences this step of activation leads to the differentiation of prosencephalic derivatives of the central nervous system (CNS) only.

Assays for the inductive power of different regions of the archenteron roof revealed a maximum of activating capacity in the prechordal plate region. This activity declines in the posterior and, more sharply, in the lateral direction. In fact, the lateral boundaries of the developed neural plate are not in direct contact with actively inducing mesoderm. These observations have led to the assumption that the primary event of induction occurs mainly along the dorsal midline and that a signal then spreads laterally within the ectodermal layer, provoking neuralization by homoiogenetic induction. The spreading of the induction within the ectoderm can be directly demonstrated by implanting a strip of ectoderm perpendicularly to the surface into the midline of the neural plate at midgastrula. Induction readily propagates into the region of the implant, which itself is not in contact with the mesoderm.

According to this idea, the lateral boundary of the neural plate is established when the neural competence of the ectoderm runs low and the spreading signal thereby becomes ineffective. In fact, a piece of competent ectoderm implanted into a region outside the neural plate of an older gastrula becomes activated, indicating that the signal readily crosses the borders of the neural plate.

The **neurectoderm** which is formed under these activating influences will develop exclusively prosencephalic structures if it is separated from further tissue interactions. The developmental fate of the activated neural ectoderm is further modulated by a second process called transformation, in which the original prosencephalic differentiation tendencies are converted into the mesencephalic, rhombencephalic, and spinal chord pathway of development. This inducing activity emanates from the notochordal region of the mesoderm, with a maximum in the caudal region. It exerts its influence up to the posterior border of the prosencephalon.

Provided that neural induction is accomplished in *Xenopus* in a similar way as in the urodeles, the behavior of the mesoderm during gastrulation offers some further explanation. Both the activating and the transforming activities move over the responding dorsal ectoderm in two consecutive waves. This is reminiscent of the movement of the two mesodermal regions defined by the spreading and the converging cell populations. Though suggestive, this does not prove that this subdivision of the early mesoderm does in fact correspond to the regionalization of the two inducing activities. Furthermore, the anterior neural plate is formed from the animal cap and the trunk neural plate from the NIMZ material. Thus, the responding tissue is already subdivided into two populations before it contacts the mesoderm. This may also contribute to their further fate.

It is also not known whether the anlage of the central nervous system is initially segregated into two compartments only, or whether several signals, perhaps modulated by the timing of the respective contacts, are used to imprint a more sophisticated pattern onto the emerging neural system. In any case, it is not reasonable to assume that the whole complex CNS structure is already reflected in the mesoderm in some way. Once a basic pattern is erected in the neural plate, self-organization within the anlage is likely to take over to work out the details.

The search for the nature of the inducing signal that is emitted from the mesoderm has a long history. In assays, either competent ectoderm obtained from late blastulae or early gastrulae is exposed in vitro to the substance under investigation or else, to minimize in vitro artifacts, a piece of insoluble material is introduced into the blastocoel of early gastrulae, where it is pressed against the ectoderm by the invo-luting cell masses during gastrulation. The formation of neural tissue is monitored either histologically or by the appearance of marker molecules indicative of neural differentiation.

The ectoderm is apparently in an unstable state during the phase of neural competence. Upon slight disturbances the ectoderm might deviate from its autonomous progression toward epidermal differentiation and enter the neurogenic pathway. Under such conditions, it is extremely difficult to define the criteria which should be met by a substance to make it eligible as a candidate for the natural inducer. In fact, the collection of substances found to be active in neural induction appears rather strange and not very informative. It comprises exotica like ectoderm killed by boiling, LiCl, basic protein from alcohol-fixed mouse kidney, cyclic AMP, Con A, and many others. Also high or low pH conditions can cause neural induction.

The supposition emerging from these observations is that rather unspecific stimuli may trigger second messenger systems in the ectodermal cells, leading to a coordinated change of intracellular conditions which then drive the development of the cells into the neural pathway. In fact, protein kinase C, a key relay in signal transduction by second messengers, is found to be activated in *Xenopus* ectodermal cells during neural induction.

Recent findings indicate that, during *Xenopus* development, anterior neural structures seem to be transformed into posterior ones when gastrulae are treated with retinoic acid. This substance influences cell differentiation and morphogenetic patterning in other systems and is known to be a direct regulator of gene activity. It is active on the *Xenopus* embryo at concentrations, comparable to those found within the embryo itself. These characteristics make it a likely candidate for the natural signal substance which induces transformation, the second step in neurogenesis. This discovery supports the notion that the two-step model for neural induction also applies for *Xenopus*.

The noninduced part of the ectoderm begins to differentiate into the two-layered embryonic epidermis at the late gastrula stage. Tonofilament bundles and desmosomes appear in the ectodermal cells at stage 12.5. Mucus-secreting vesicular cells begin to form at this stage and become functional at stage 17. Ciliated cells insert into the outer, **epithelial layer of epidermal ectoderm** from the inner, **sensorial layer of epidermal ectoderm** at stage 18.

Morphogenesis of the Neural Tube

The most obvious changes in cell shape after neural induction occur in the **sensorial layer of the neurectoderm** from stage 12 onwards. The cells lateral to the dorsal midline elongate to form a columnar epithelium, a process in which the whole neural plate becomes thickened and bulges slightly (PLATES 20; 21). Since the outer ectodermal cells do not yet exhibit a recognizable change in shape, and continuity is preserved in both ectodermal layers, the two layers must slide past each other and the cells of the inner layer lateral to the neural plate must become thinner by stretching to compensate for the dorsal thickening.

The response to induction is not confined, however, to the inner ectodermal cell layer. An antigen (Epi 1) appears on the surface of the superficial ectoderm cells as they differentiate into epidermis at midgastrula stages. Its expression is inhibited in the neural plate area indicating that the superficial cell layer responds to induction as well, but in a different way.

The neural plate begins to narrow particularly in the central and posterior region of the embryo at stage 15 (PLATE 28). The anterolateral edge begins to thicken at stage 16 (PLATE 27). The **neurocoel** forms when the **neural tube** closes at stage 20 (PLATE 33). The mechanism of neural tube closure is an interesting example of coordinated morphogenetic movements.

As described above, the neural plate has been patterned in the anterior-posterior direction by the activating and transforming influences of the mesoderm. The discrete modes of behavior of the different regions of the neural plate during neural tube closure reveal a pattern in the mediolateral direction as well.

In a narrow strip along the midline of the neural plate the cells of the sensorial layer do not participate in the columnarization thus forming a shallow groove. These cells are derived from the dorsal NIMZ of the early gastrula and have been pushed anteriorly by convergent extension. They form a separate compartment within the neural plate as they do not intermingle with the lateral neural plate cells, thus maintaining a sharp lateral boundary. Apparently, the emergence of this cell population does not depend on induction by the underlying notochord. They already exhibit a predisposition for their distinct behavior at the onset of gastrulation. These cells might be determined by the tangential spreading of an inductive signal from the noninvoluted IMZ at the early gastrula phase. Because of its distinct properties this region is distinguished from the rest of the neural plate by designating it as the **notoplate** (PLATES 21; 23).

At the onset of neural fold formation at stage 15 the superficial cells of the notoplate form typical bottle cells by apical constriction, thereby contributing to

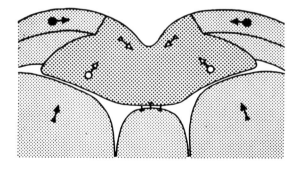

Fig. 9.3. Diagrammatic portrayal of five possible sources of mechanical force affecting the progress of neurulation. Autonomous forces acting within the neural plate include: apical contraction of the median superficial ectoderm zone (*open double arrows*) and cellular elongation in the lateral wall (*open circled arrows*). Extrinsic forces include: elongation of myotome cells (*solid double arrows*), medial convergence of epidermis (*solid circled arrows*), and the adhesive relationship between notochord and neural plate. (Schroeder 1970)

the deepening of the **neural groove** (PLATES 27; 28). They remain in close contact with the cells of the ectodermal deep layer, until the two layers eventually interdigitate to form the unilayered floor of the neural tube.

Microdissection experiments reveal that notoplate and notochord are attached to each other quite firmly throughout the process of neural fold formation, whereas the lateral regions of the neural plate may be easily lifted off from the underlying mesoderm. This attachment may link notochord extension and the generation of the keyhole shape of the neural plate, the posterior region of the latter being stretched mechanically by the extending notochord. The keyhole shape of the neural plate anticipates the distribution of neural and neural crest material along the body axis, both decreasing in amount posteriorly.

Some observations in *Xenopus* indicate that the conditions may not be quite as simple as described above. Notochordless embryos, generated by UV treatment of the zygote, form a well-shaped neural plate, and in explants the ectoderm derived from the NIMZ exhibits autonomous convergent extension in the absence of the underlying notochord. Perhaps this autonomous behavior of the notoplate region and the mechanical influence of notochord stretching act synergistically in shaping the neural plate.

As may be recognized from the corresponding cross-sections, the paraxial mesoderm is gradually lifted above the level of the notochord (cf. PLATES 28 and 30). As notoplate and notochord remain connected, this contributes to a further deepening of the neural groove and a lifting of the lateral neural plate (Fig. 9.3).

As neural tube formation progresses a group of superficial cells lateral to the bottle cells forms the roof plate of the neural tube, which is later overlaid by lateral ectoderm migrating medially. The columnar inner cells of the lateral neural plate tilt dorsomedially and come to constitute the lateral walls of the neural tube, from which later most of the neural tissue is generated (PLATES 28; 30; 33), (Fig. 9.4).

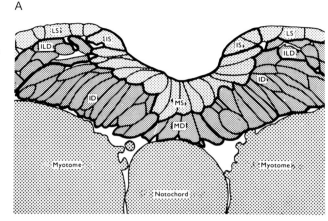

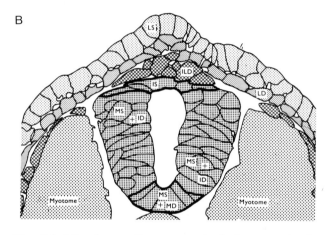

Fig. 9.4. Morphogenetic movements during neural tube closure between stage 16 and stage 22. The invaginating neural plate has been divided into the following regions: *LS* lateral superficial; *IS* intermediate superficial; *MS* median superficial; *LD* lateral deep; *ILD* intermedio-lateral deep; *ID* intermediate deep; *MD* median deep. **A** shows the regions before, **B** illustrates the rearrangement of these regions after neural tube closure. (Schroeder 1970)

Still further outward, the lateralmost margin of the deep layer of the neural plate does not participate in this movement and is not integrated into the neural tube. Signs of a separation of this cell group from the bulk of neurogenic material are first seen at stage 15/16. These cells are the precursors of **neural crest** cells, which later display migratory behavior

Neural crest cells and their descendants can then be traced throughout the life of such a chimera.

Neural crest material may be histologically distinguished from neural plate material proper, when the folding of the neural tube begins at stage 15/16. Due to their active participation in neural folding the neural plate cells are oriented toward the dorsal midline, whereas the neural crest cells are not arranged in any special order. This is particularly obvious in the head region, where neural crest material represents an appreciable amount of the lateral neurectoderm (PLATE 27). Rostrally, the crest material extends up to the posterior boundary of the eye anlage, the prosencephalic region being free of neural crest (Fig. 10.3). Much less neural crest material is seen in the trunk region (PLATE 28).

It has been suggested that neural induction plays a role in the determination of neural crest migratory behavior. When the neural competence of the ectoderm fades, the competence for neural crest formation persists for some time during which the cells are exposed to the transforming signal emanating from the central neural plate region. Thus, neural crest material forms at the neural plate boundary at the end of the period of neural competence.

The migratory behavior of neural crest cells and their pathways of migration differ considerably in the head and trunk region. Scanning electron microscopy of a stage 16 embryo reveals that the head region contains a set of three major segments of neural crest material, separated from each other by grooves. The segments become more compact in the following stages, and at stage 19, when the neural tube is still open, the neural crest cell masses begin to migrate as coherent streams of cells.

One stream, the mandibular crest segment, which originates from the mesencephalic region, moves ventrally and curves toward the eye anlage at stage 21–22. By stage 24 the eye anlage is completely surrounded by these cells. The hyoid segment originates from the anterior rhombencephalic region. Cells of this segment descend rostrally from the otic vesicle to join the mesoderm of the hyoid arch. The branchial crest segment migrates posteriorly from

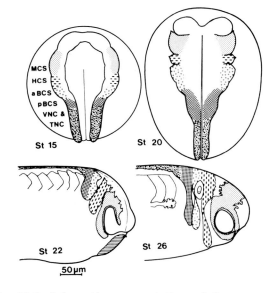

Fig. 10.1. Schematic representation of the appearance and the migration of the neural crest material at different stages. *MCS* Mandibular crest segment; *HCS* hyoid crest segment; *aBCS* anterior branchial crest segment; *pBCS* posterior branchial crest segment; *VNC* and *TNC* vagal and trunkal neural crest. (Sadaghiani and Thibaud 1987)

the otic vesicle and divides into an anterior and posterior portion, which meet in the future branchial region at stages 24–26. Figure 10.1 gives a summary of neural crest migration in the head region.

In the cross-section of stage 23, neural crest material extends from its site of origin to the dorsal side of the eye anlage (PLATE 38B). At stage 26 the eye is completely surrounded by this material (PLATE 41). The lateral border of the eye vesicle is in close contact with the epidermis and free of neural crest material. As neural crest material has been found to inhibit lens formation in the ectoderm, the surrounding of the eye cup with neural crest material has been considered to be of importance for the proper positioning of the lens, which forms at stage 27 (PLATE 42).

In the trunk region, the neural crest material comes to lie dorsal to the neural tube during tube closure. Crest migration does not begin before stage 28, much later than in the head region. Using the trans-

plantation method, cells have been observed to move along three defined routes: dorsally into the fin, ventrally along the somite-neural tube and -notochord border, and to a lesser extent laterally along the somite-epidermis border (Fig. 10.2). In contrast to those in the head region the trunk crest cells migrate individually and not as a coherent mass. These events cannot be seen in the stages presented in the plates.

Much work has been devoted to defining the signals and substrates which might direct neural crest migration into these defined routes. It is obvious from the above description that the cells tend to use preexisting clefts between the tissues as pathways for their initial migration. Components of the extracellular matrix such as fibronectin and tenascin have been postulated to be involved in the migration. On the way to their target sites the migrating

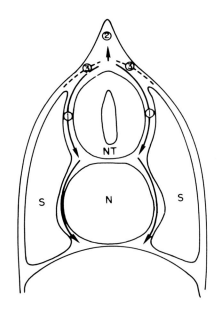

Fig. 10.2. Schematic diagram illustrating the pathways of neural crest cell migration in the trunk of *Xenopus: 1* a ventral pathway between neural tube (*NT*) and somite (*S*), notochord (*N*) and somite, and along the dorsal mesentery; *2* a dorsal pathway into the fin; and *3* a minor lateral pathway (observed in *borealis/laevis* chimerae and blastomere-injected embryos) between somite and epidermis. (Krotoski et al. 1988)

crest cells become sequentially induced to form certain cell types. These events have been extensively analyzed in systems other than *Xenopus*.

Placodes

The placodes comprise a set of local thickenings within the sensorial layer of the cephalic ectoderm. They represent the anlagen for the adenohypophysis, the olfactory organ, the lens, the ear, the lateral line system, and the cranial ganglia.

Analysis of their development in amphibians other than *Xenopus* has led to the assumption that they may be traced back to a common origin. A band of thickened ectoderm, the "primitive placodal thickening" surrounds the neural plate and neural crest area of the neurula. The anlagen of the placodes are situated within this band (Fig. 10.3).

The position of this band at the outermost boundary of the neural plate suggests that its emergence is related to the processes of neuroinduction. A mechanism similar to that giving rise to the neural crest is proposed. In fact, a strip of competent ectoderm transplanted vertically into the neural plate receives a signal to form neural and placodal tissue by homoiogenetic induction. Competence for placode formation persists considerably longer than neural competence.

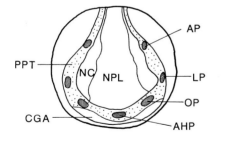

Fig. 10.3. The placodal anlagen in the *Rana* embryo. *NPL* Definite neural plate; *NC* neural crest; *PPT* primitive placodal thickening; *CGA* cement gland anlage. The placodal anlagen are: *AP* auditory placode; *LP* lens placode; *OP* olfactory placode; *AHP* adenohypophyseal placode. (After Knouff 1935)

The fact that the primitive band of placodal thickening later disappears locally in the regions between the placodes indicates that further signals are required for the differentiation and proper positioning of the individual placodes. A system of successive inductions has been proposed, in which the head endoderm provides the primary signal as it moves underneath the placodal ectoderm during gastrulation. The successive contacts with head mesodermal regions during gastrulation enhance and modify the signal. Neural crest material may play an important role in delimiting the site of placode formation.

Only recently have selected aspects of placode formation been investigated in the *Xenopus* embryo. The primary band of placodal thickening is difficult to discern in *Xenopus*. A recent analysis of **lens** formation in *Xenopus* yielded results which are in accordance with the view of placode formation outlined above. This view disagrees with classical concepts in which the main emphasis was placed on an inductive influence of the eye vesicle.

An indication of the early **olfactory placode** is seen in the anteriormost ectoderm at stage 23. The placode is more pronounced at stage 26 (PLATE 39). Lens formation is obvious at stage 27 (PLATE 42), and the formation of the **ear placode** and its invagination to form the ear vesicle is depicted in PLATE 43.

Cement Gland

The **cement gland** is a most conspicuous epidermal differentiation of the early embryo. The first indication of the presumptive gland region is an accumulation of pigment at the anteriormost border of the neural plate at stage 15. The gland begins to protrude at stage 23 and becomes functional in secreting mucous "cement" at stage 28.

Histologically, the prospective gland becomes apparent at stage 19/20 (PLATE 31). At this stage, the anlage begins to segregate from the ectodermal layer. The cells become columnar and densely packed.

In the transverse section of stage 23 one can recognize that the glandular cells proper arise from the outer epidermal layer, while the sensorial layer of the ectoderm is transformed into the very thin basal layer of the gland (PLATE 38). The gland is also a prominent feature in the transverse sections through the head region from stage 20 onwards.

Some data on the developmental origin of this structure are available. At stage 10 the whole outer layer of early gastrula ectoderm may be induced to form gland epithelium by exposing the isolate to 10 mM ammonium chloride. Competence for this reaction is lost by stage 12/13. It may be inferred from these results that in situ induction occurs at this time. The ectodermal area in which the cement gland eventually forms is exceptional in that it remains in close contact with the endoderm after gastrulation with no intervening mesoderm. This arrangement is considered to be important for the proper positioning of the cement gland anlage.

Mesodermal Derivatives

Pronephros

The pronephros develops from the lateral plate mesoderm adjacent to the axial mesoderm. At stage 20 the double-layered sheet of lateral plate mesoderm lines the endodermal yolk mass (PLATE 33). The outer layer represents the **somatic** (or parietal) **layer** and the inner layer represents the **splanchnic** (or visceral) **layer**. At stage 21 a thickening of the somatic layer is visible at the border between the head and the trunk (PLATES 38; 39; 41A; 43). This is the first indication of the **prophric anlage**. By stage 24 the cells of this region have become columnar in shape and appear bent and bottle-shaped. The organ anlage has become completely segregated from the surrounding mesoderm by stage 27.

The pronephric duct is then formed by local recruitment of cells from the posterior lateral plate, with no long-range cell movement being involved. The segregation of the pronephric duct propagates as a wave from anterior to posterior. Like the somitic segmentation process, this wave is of the cinematic type, as it is insensitive to local disturbances. Pronephric duct formation in *Xenopus* is radically different from that seen in urodeles, where the duct consists of cells that have emigrated from the pronephric anlage, and elongation of the duct is achieved by cell rearrangement.

Heart

In the dorsolateral portion of the anterior mesodermal mantle the prospective heart mesoderm is localized in two portions on either side of the prechordal plate. At the onset of neurulation, prospective heart mesoderm begins to move laterally along the anterior edge of the mesodermal mantle. During the late neurula stages, the two heart anlagen fuse ventrally posterior to the cement gland, where they give rise to the endocardium at stage 27/28. Only at these late stages can the **heart anlage** be safely discerned in the plates (PLATES 39; 42A).

Explantation experiments have indicated that heart mesoderm specification occurs during the midgastrula and late gastrula stages. An inductive influence of the head endoderm is required for heart formation in the urodeles. This influence seems not to be necessary in *Xenopus*.

Endodermal Derivatives

At stage 20 (PLATE 31) the earliest indication of the subdivision of the archenteron into the **foregut**, **midgut**, and **hindgut** is visible. The stretching of the embryo, which begins at this stage, shifts the yolk mass dorsally. The median portion of the archenteron forms the slit-shaped archenteric canal (PLATE 36). From the foregut the **visceral pouches** and the **oral evagination** develop. The visceral pouches evaginate toward opposing thickenings of the sensorial layer of the ectoderm, which develop simultaneously. Intimate contacts between the visceral pouches and the ectoderm are established from stage 24 onwards. The branchial membranes consisting of ecto- and endodermal material will finally be formed in these zones. Neural crest material invades the region between the visceral pouches and forms the **branchial arches**. The mandibular arch is formed anterior to the first visceral pouch, the hyoid arch separates the first and second visceral pouch, and the first branchial arch separates the second and third visceral pouch (PLATES 39; 40).

The oral evagination of the foregut begins with a slight bulge at stage 20 (PLATE 31) and forms a wedge-shaped endodermal protrusion at stage 23 (PLATE 36) when it contacts the **stomodeal-hypophyseal anlage,** a thickening in the opposing sensorial layer of the ectoderm. At later stages, not included in this atlas, the hypophyseal anlage separates from the epidermal thickening of the stomodeum. The stomodeum fuses with the endodermal evagination, which ruptures and forms the mouth opening.

A further differentiation of the foregut is the **liver diverticulum**. It first appears as a ventral extension of the anterior part of the archenteron at stages 15/16 (PLATE 26) and gradually deepens (PLATE 31). This extension becomes dorsoventrally compressed at stage 23 (PLATE 36) and forms a very narrow slit at stage 26. Later at stage 33 the anterior wall of the liver rudiment will bulge forward to form the primary hepatic cavity.

In stage 23 the gut is seen to extend beyond the original blastopore into the tail region (PLATE 37). At stage 26 (PLATE 39B) the postanal gut extends into the tail bud, and the posterior midgut has widened. At later stages the midgut will bend ventrally to meet the ectodermal rudiment of the cloaca, whereas the postanal gut will disappear.

References

Reviews

SAHA, M. S., SPANN, C. L. & GRAINGER, R. M. (1989). Embryonic lens induction: more than meets the optic vesicle. *Cell Differ. Dev.* **28**, 153-172.

JACOBSON, A. G. & SATER, A. K. (1988). Features of embryonic induction. *Development* **104**, 341-359.

WINKLBAUER, R. (1989). Development of the lateral line system in *Xenopus*. *Progress in Neurobiology* **32**, 181-206.

Original Communications

BRUN, R. B. (1981). The movement of the prospective eye vesicles from the neural plate into the neural fold in *Ambystoma mexicanum* and *Xenopus laevis*. *Dev. Biol.* **88**, 192-199.

EPPERLEIN, H. H., HALFTER, W. & TUCKER, R. P. (1988). The distribution of fibronectin and tenascin along migratory pathways of the neural crest in the trunk of amphibian embryos. *Development* **103**, 743-756.

FOX, H. & HAMILTON, L. (1964). Origin of the pronephric duct in *Xenopus laevis*. *Arch. Biol. (Liège)* **75**, 245-251.

KLEIN, S. L. & GRAZIADEI, P. P. C. (1983). The differentiation of the olfactory placode in *Xenopus laevis*: a light and electron microscope study. *J. Comp. Neurol.* **217**, 17-30.

KNOUFF, R. A. (1935). The developmental pattern of ectodermal placodes in *Rana pipiens*. *J. Comp. Neurol.* **62**, 17-71.

KROTOSKI, D. M., FRASER, S. E. & BRONNER-FRASER, M. (1988). Mapping of neural crest pathways in *Xenopus laevis* using inter- and intra-specific cell markers. *Dev. Biol.* **127**, 119-132.

LYERLA, T. A. & PELIZZARI, J. J. (1973). Histological development of the cement gland in *Xenopus laevis*: a light microscopic study. *J. Morphol.* **141**, 491-495.

PICARD, J. J. (1975). *Xenopus laevis* cement gland as an experimental model for embryonic differentiation. I. In vitro stimulation of differentiation by ammonium chloride. *J. Embryol. Exp. Morphol.* **33,4**, 957-967.

PICARD, J. J. (1975). *Xenopus laevis* cement gland as an experimental model for embryonic differentiation. II. The competence of embryonic cells. *J. Embryol. Exp. Morphol.* **33,4**, 969-978.

PICARD, J. J. (1976). Ultrastructure of the cement gland of *Xenopus laevis*. *J. Morphol.* **148**, 193-197.

POOLE, T. J. & STEINBERG, M. S. (1984). Different modes of pronephric duct origin among vertebrates. *Scanning Electron Microscopy* **1**, 475-482.

SADAGHIANI, B. & THIEBAUD, C. H. (1987). Neural crest development in the *Xenopus laevis* embryo, studied by interspecific transplantation and scanning electron microscopy. *Dev. Biol.* **124**, 91-110.

SATER, A. K. & JACOBSON, A. G. (1989). The specification of heart mesoderm occurs during gastrulation in *Xenopus laevis*. *Development* **105**, 821-830.

The Histology

Histological Procedures

For the advanced stages of oogenesis and all embryonic stages, Romeis fixative was used. This fixative allows a good overall preservation of the embryonic structures with little shrinkage or swelling. For the stages of early oogenesis paraformaldehyde-glutaraldehyde rendered a better preservation of the more delicate intracellular structures.

All specimens were embedded in glycol methacrylate. Resin embedding is decisive for good quality sections and is superior to the conventional wax procedures. Sectioning with Ralph glass knives was convenient and gave excellent results.

To illustrate the most relevant features of the individual developmental stages, different staining methods had to be applied. For the stages of oogenesis and early cleavage, staining procedures were chosen which emphasize intracellular details. To visualize the mitochondrial aggregates in early oocytes acid fuchsin/methylene blue staining was used, azure B was applied to demonstrate cytoplasmic structures other than yolk, and azofuchsin/aniline blue/orange G was used to illustrate the overall arrangement of the intracellular structures. At the later stages of embryonic development, the shape and the arrangement of the individual cells were regarded as the most important features. DNA and polysaccharide components were stained using brilliant cresyl blue as a Schiff's reagent. The nuclei and the cell borders were thus stained producing the graphical appearance of the plates from the later stages.

To achieve the desired resolution the stained sections were photographed at high magnification, which meant that up to eight shots had to be taken to cover one section. The individual negatives were printed separately and then assembled in a composite plate. This procedure explains the slightly different shadings within some of the plates.

The legends accompanying the photographic plates are headed by three boxes. The first box gives the plate number and the stage of the oocyte or embryo shown. The staging of the embryos was carried out according to Nieuwkoop and Faber's normal table.

In some cases external and internal criteria did not match exactly and a compromise was chosen.

The arrows in the second box indicate the direction of the embryonic axes in the section.

In the third box the plane of sectioning is indicated as a dashed line in drawings taken from Nieuwkoop and Faber's normal table. The drawings represent external views of the embryos from different angles. If a suitable drawing of a certain stage was not available in the normal table, a drawing of a stage close to the one on the photograph was chosen. Strictly sagittal sections of later embryos are difficult to obtain because the embryonic axis tends to bend slightly. The plane of sectioning through bent embryos is indicated by a curved dashed line in the drawing of a straight embryo.

Fixation Procedures

Paraformaldehyde-Glutaraldehyde Fixative

Specimens were fixed in 2% paraformaldehyde and 1% glutaraldehyde in 0.05 M phosphate buffer for 5 h at room temperature. They were rinsed in buffer twice for 10 min and then dehydrated in graded ethanol.

Romeis Fixative (Romeis 1968)

Embryos were fixed with Romeis fixative (25 ml saturated mercuric chloride; 20 ml 5% trichloro-acetic acid; 15 ml 37% formaldehyde) for 1−3 h at room temperature and then transferred to 100% ethanol for 2 h with one change.

Embedding and Sectioning

Glycol Methacrylate

The fixed and dehydrated objects were infiltrated in 50% Technovit 7100 infiltration solution in ethanol for 1 h and left in 100% Technovit 7100 infiltration solution overnight. Polymerization was carried out at room temperature. Technovit 7100 is a glycol methacrylate derivate sold by Kulzer and Co., 6393

Wehrheim, FRG. 3–5 µm sections were obtained with Ralph glass knives.

Plexiglass
Objects were infiltrated in 50% dichloromethane (CH_2Cl_2) in ethanol for 2 h and in 100% CH_2Cl_2 for another 2 h. They were then transferred to 24% plexiglass (Röhm GmbH, 6100 Darmstadt, FRG) in CH_2Cl_2 and stored in an airtight container for 1 week before the CH_2Cl_2 was allowed to evaporate. 1–5 µm sections were obtained with Ralph glass knives. The plastic was removed by CH_2Cl_2, and the sections were rehydrated by a series of graded ethanol. (Hausen 1988)

Removal of Mercury Precipitates (Romeis 1968)

The dry sections were treated with an alcoholic iodine potassium iodide solution (2% iodine, 3% potassium iodide in 90% ethanol) for 2 min, washed in 0.25% sodium thiosulfate for 15 min and thoroughly rinsed in distilled water.

Staining Procedures

All dyes were obtained from Chroma Gesellschaft, 7000 Stuttgart, FRG.
Unless stated differently the stained sections were left to dry at room temperature and mounted in Entellan (Merck, 6100 Darmstadt, FRG).

AAO (azofuchsin/aniline blue/orange G triple staining)
The sections were treated as follows: 1% azofuchsin in 1% acetic acid for 14 min; distilled water; 0.5% aniline blue, 2% orange G in 8% acetic acid (boiled) for 14 min; distilled water; 0.5% aniline blue in water for 10 min; distilled water.

TB (toluidine blue in borax; after Tourte et al. 1984)
The sections were stained in 1% toluidine blue in 1% borax for 30 s.

AFMB (acid fuchsin/methylene blue double staining)
The sections were stained in 2% acid fuchsin in 5% phenol (60 °C) for 30–40 min, 0.06% methylene blue for 2 s, 0.3% methylene blue for 3 min, and then rinsed in water or differentiated in absolute ethanol.

Azure B
The sections were stained in 0.025% azure B in 0.1 M citric acid/phosphate buffer (pH 4) for 3–4 h.

PD (*p*-phenylenediamine)
The plexiglass sections were treated as follows: 100 mM periodic acid for 30 min; distilled water; 0.1% p-phenylenediamine (recrystallized) for 30 min; distilled water; graded ethanol series. They were then left to dry and mounted in glycerine.

BCB (brilliant cresyl blue SO_2, combined Feulgen and PAS reaction after Kasten 1960)
The sections were treated as follows: 0.5% periodic acid in 50% phosphoric acid for 14 min; 2 changes of distilled water; 0.75 g brilliant cresyl blue in a solution of 12.5 ml 1N HCl and 0.6 g $Na_2S_2O_5$ brought to 100 ml for 1 h; 3 changes of sulfite water (15 g $Na_2S_2O_5$, 15 ml 1N HCl brought to 300 ml); running tap water for 30 min.

References

HAUSEN, P. (1988). A new method to prepare sections from amphibian embryos for immunohistology. *Z. Naturforsch.* **43c**, 765-768.
KASTEN, F. H. (1960). The chemistry of Schiff's reagent. *Int. Rev. Cytol.* **10**, 1-100.
ROMEIS, B. (1968). Mikroskopische Technik, 16. Aufl., München, Wien: Oldenbourg.
TOURTE, M., MIGNOTTE, F., MOUNOLU, J. C. (1984). Heterogeneous distribution and replication activity of mitochondria in *Xenopus laevis*. *Eur. J. Cell Biol.* **34**, 171-178.

The Plates

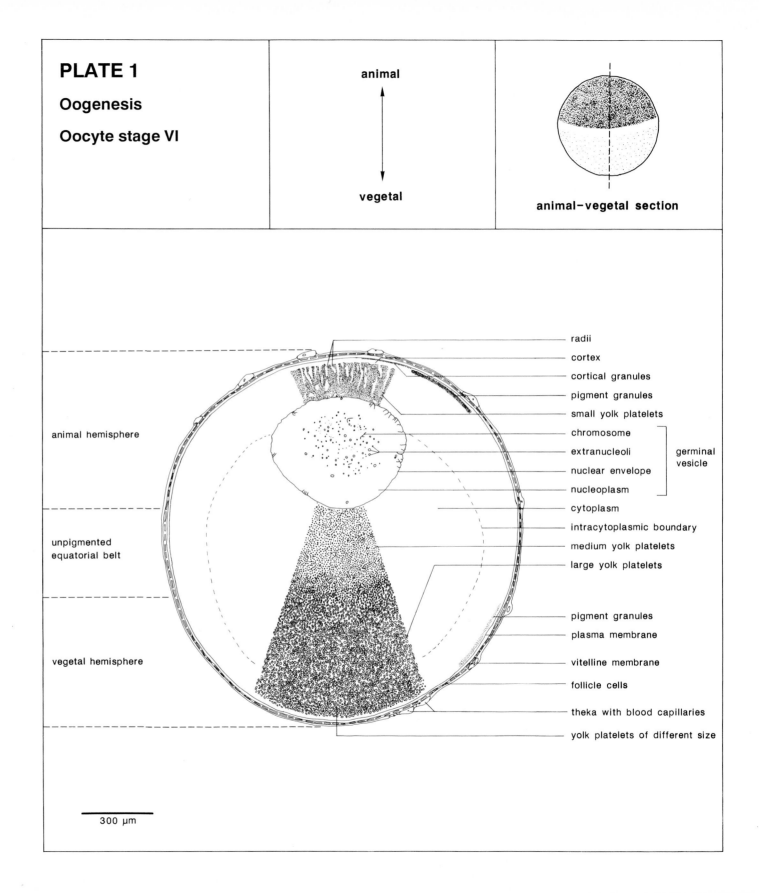

PLATE 1

Oogenesis

Oocyte stage VI

animal

vegetal

animal–vegetal section

radii

cortex

cortical granules

pigment granules

small yolk platelets

chromosome

extranucleoli

nuclear envelope

nucleoplasm

germinal vesicle

animal hemisphere

cytoplasm

intracytoplasmic boundary

medium yolk platelets

large yolk platelets

unpigmented equatorial belt

pigment granules

plasma membrane

vitelline membrane

vegetal hemisphere

follicle cells

theka with blood capillaries

yolk platelets of different size

300 µm

The Fully Grown Oocyte

(Staining: AAO)

PLATE 1

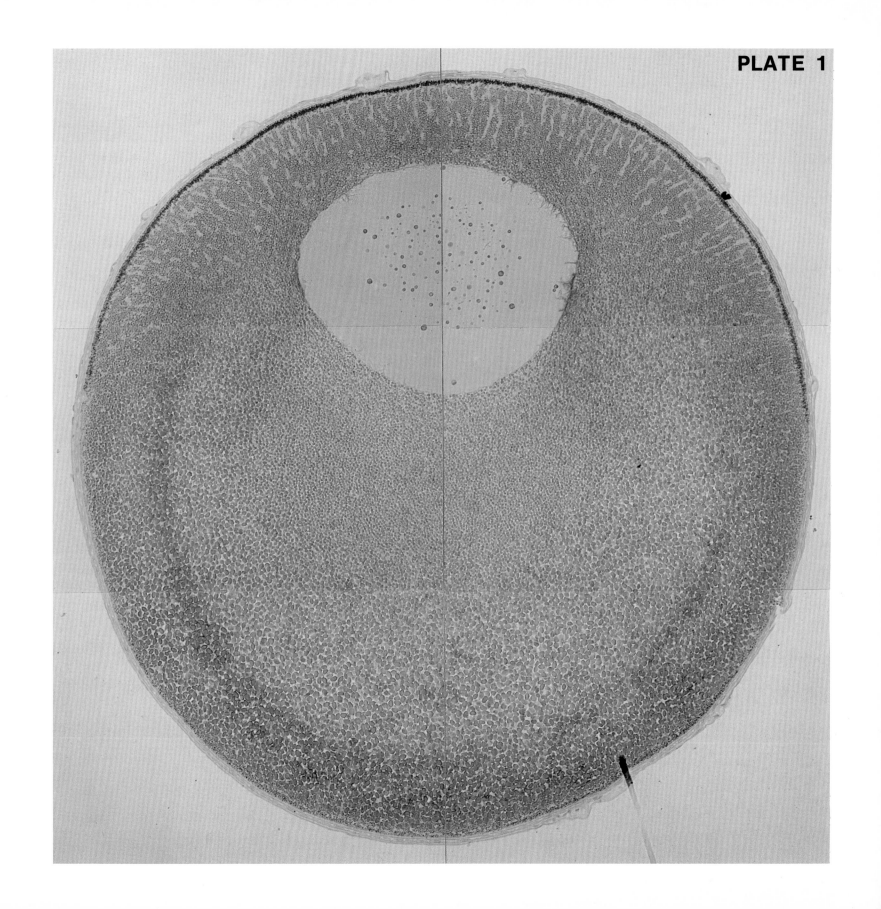

PLATE 2

Oogenesis

Premeiotic Oogonia and Oocytes in Early Meiotic Prophase

A Primary Oogonium

The ovary of premetamorphic tadpoles consists of two lobe-shaped ridges, the section through one of which is shown. The primary oogonium at the tip of the ridge is distinguished from the surrounding somatic cells by its large size, the lobed shape of the nucleus, and the uneven and condensed appearance of the chromatin. (Staining: azure B; magnification: 820x)

B Mitochondrial Aggregate in a Primary Oogonium

A primary oogonium is situated between nests of leptotene stage oocytes in the growing ovary of a young frog. The lobed nucleus and the mitochondrial mass are the most conspicuous features of the oogonium. The mitochondrial aggregate appears dark red to violet after staining with acid fuchsin/methylene blue. (Staining: AFMB; magnification: 820x)

C Secondary Oogonia

A nest of secondary oogonia undergoes synchronous mitoses, indicating their intercellular coupling by cytoplasmic bridges. (Staining: azure B; magnification: 820x)

D Preleptotene Oocytes

Preleptotene oocytes show more compact and rounded nuclei with prominent nucleoli. The nuclei contain conspicuous, unstained bodies of unknown nature. These bodies are prevalent in all oocyte nuclei up to early diplotene and then disappear. (Staining: AFMB; magnification: 820x)

E Leptotene Oocytes

A nest of oocytes in the leptotene stage is shown. The chromatin is further condensed. The mitochondrial aggregates point toward the center of the nest, indicating the cell polarity. (Staining: AFMB; magnification: 820x)

F Pachytene Oocytes

The homologous chromatides are aligned in synaptonemal complexes visible as threadlike structures.

The polarity of the oocytes is expressed by several morphological features. The mitochondrial aggregate is located in the cytoplasm next to the region of the nuclear membrane from which the synaptonemal complexes extend into the nucleus. The nucleoli are situated in the chromatin-free nuclear cap region, which is the site of ribosomal DNA amplification. Two cells at the center of the photograph display these features best. (Staining: AFMB; magnification: 820x)

G Early Diplotene Oocytes

The nuclear cap has expanded, the extranucleoli begin to form, and the synaptonemal complexes decondense. The position of the mitochondrial aggregate and the arrangement of the structures within the nucleus are indicative of the cell polarity. The cells begin to enlarge, the cytoplasm attains a light blue staining probably due to the accumulation of RNA. (Staining: AFMB; magnification: 820x)

H Stage I Oocyte

Within the nucleus the chromosomes have assumed the lampbrush configuration. Extranucleoli are sequestered at the outer border of the nucleus. From this stage onwards the acidophilic blue staining in the cytoplasm is more intense than in the nucleus, indicating a relative increase of the cytoplasmic RNA concentration. The mitochondrial aggregate is condensed into the spherical Balbiani body (violet color). The oocyte is surrounded by a loose layer of follicle cells. (Staining: AFMB; magnification: 400x)

Photograph **A** was taken from an ovary of a stage 55 tadpole, photographs **B-H** were taken from ovaries of frogs that were 2–6 months old.

PLATE 2

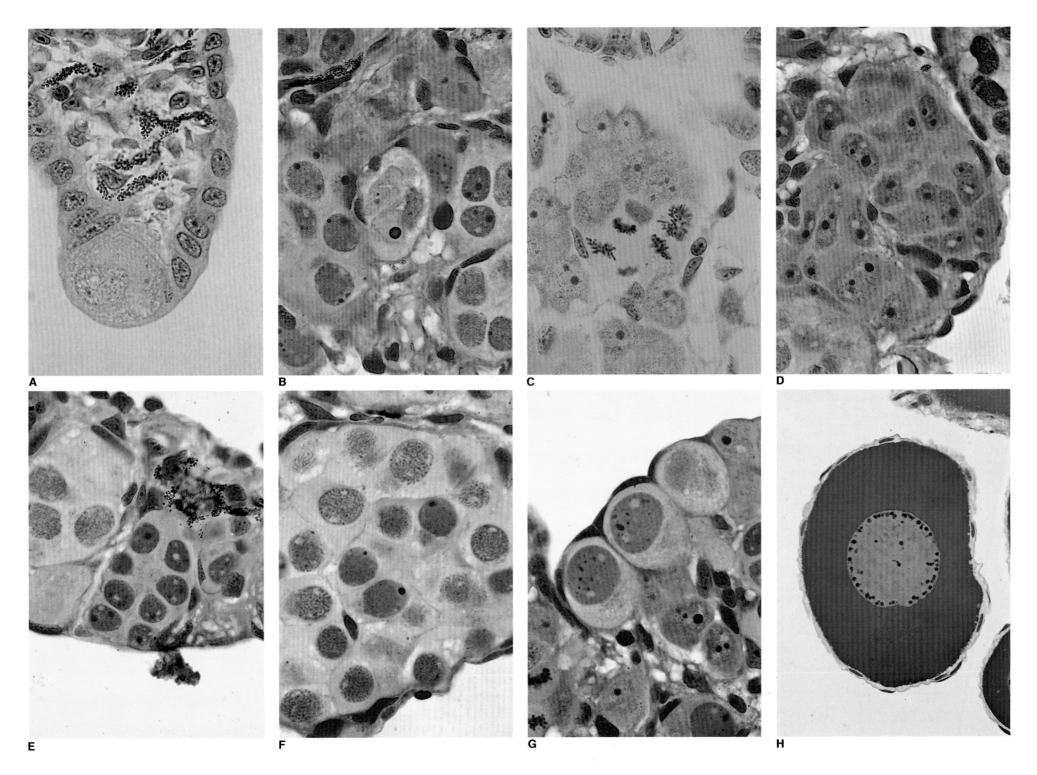

PLATE 3

Oogenesis

Oocytes Stages I-IV

A Late Stage I Oocytes

The nucleus shows a slight depression in the vicinity of the Balbiani body . Nucleoli are displaced from this site. The follicle cell layer is dense. (Staining: AFMB; magnification: 170x)

B Early Stage II Oocyte

The nuclear envelope is lobed. Extranucleoli are scattered throughout the nucleoplasm with a preference for the outer regions. The Balbiani body is segregated into fragments. One portion of the fragments begins to surround the nucleus and to disperse into the cytoplasm. The other portion of the fragments is transported toward the future vegetal pole of the oocyte. Unstained lipid deposits begin to appear in the outer region of the cytoplasm. (Staining: AFMB; magnification: 170x)

C Late Stage II Oocyte

Lampbrush chromosomes have gathered in the center of the nucleus, the extranucleoli are localized more to the margin. The Balbiani body is completely fragmented, a portion of the fragments has settled in the vegetal cortical region. Lipid deposits have shifted from the cortical position to the interior. The oocyte is surrounded by a layer of follicle cells and the theca layer, which contains blood capillaries. (Staining: AFMB; magnification: 200x)

D Stage III Oocyte, Early Vitellogenesis

The lampbrush chromosomes begin to condense. Nucleoli are more variable in size and more evenly scattered within the nucleoplasm. The polarized localization of material from the Balbiani body is pronounced. The yolk platelets are quite uniform in size and evenly positioned in the outer portion of the cytoplasm. Lipid deposits have become sparse. A layer of cortical granules lines the plasma membrane within the cortex. The collagenase used to isolate this oocyte has removed the ovarian tissue, including the follicle layer, leaving only the vitelline membrane around the oocyte. (Staining: AFMB; magnification: 200x)

E Stage IV Oocyte, Midvitellogenesis

Pigment granules appear in the cortex beneath the cortical granules around the whole circumference of the oocyte. Pigmentation indicates a difference in thickness of the cortex in the animal and the vegetal hemisphere. The radii begin to develop in the animal hemisphere. Yolk platelets in the vegetal region are larger than in the animal region. The material derived from the cortical portion of Balbiani body fragments forms a thin, pink layer between the pigment of the vegetal cortex and the vegetal yolk. (Staining: AFMB; magnification: 140x)

F Cortical Granules in Stage II and IV Oocytes

The cortical granules show up in bright yellow with this fluorescent staining. In the stage II oocyte (*upper specimen*) the cortical granules are seen in the peripheral cytoplasm. In the stage IV oocyte (*lower specimen*) they have aligned in a broad layer between pigment granules and plasma membrane. (Embedding medium: Plexiglass; staining: PD; magnification: 360x)

G Cortical Granules in Stage VI Oocyte

They form a single layer in the vegetal cortex of a stage VI oocyte. (Embedding medium: Plexiglass; staining: PD; magnification: 250x)

The oocytes of the different stages were obtained from adult females.

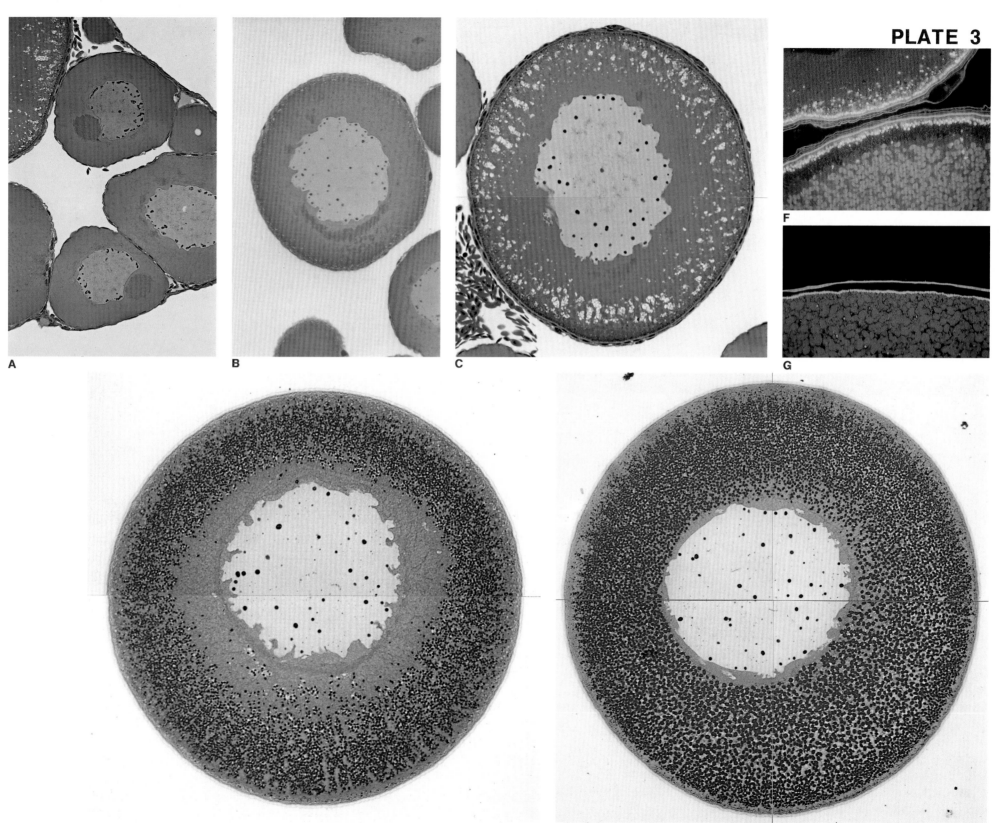

PLATE 3

A

B

C

F

G

D

E

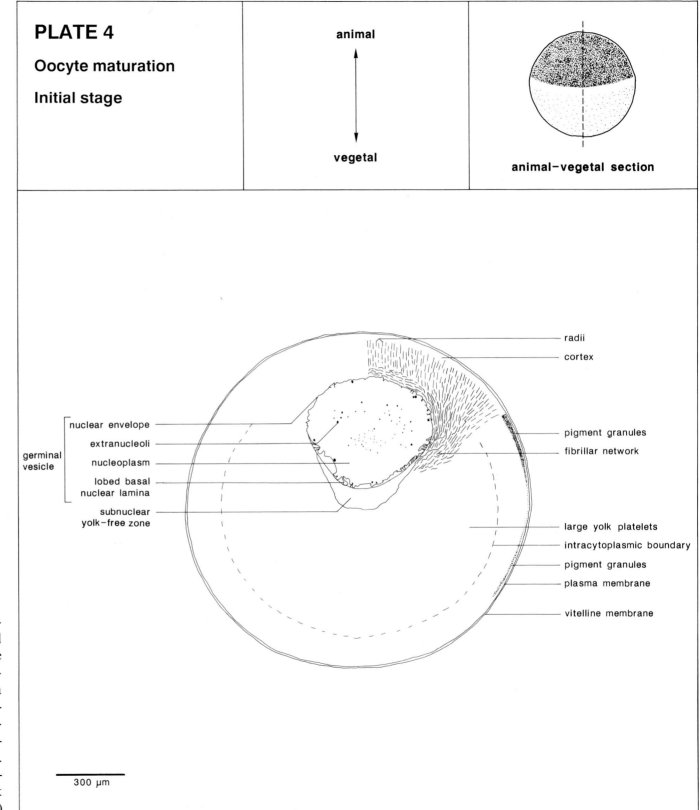

PLATE 4

Oocyte maturation

Initial stage

animal

vegetal

animal–vegetal section

radii

cortex

nuclear envelope

extranucleoli

pigment granules

fibrillar network

nucleoplasm

germinal
vesicle

lobed basal
nuclear lamina

subnuclear
yolk-free zone

large yolk platelets

intracytoplasmic boundary

pigment granules

plasma membrane

vitelline membrane

300 µm

Initiation of Germinal Vesicle Breakdown

The oocyte was incubated with 10 µg/ml progesterone for 4 h prior to fixation. The germinal vesicle contains numerous extranucleoli, the larger ones are localized more to the outer region, the smaller ones more to the center. As a first sign of the onset of germinal vesicle breakdown the basal nuclear envelope is lobed. A subnuclear yolk-free zone, known to contain fascicles of microtubuli, extends into the cytoplasm. The growth of this zone seems to affect the arrangement of the radii and the fibrillar network within the animal hemisphere. (Staining: azure B)

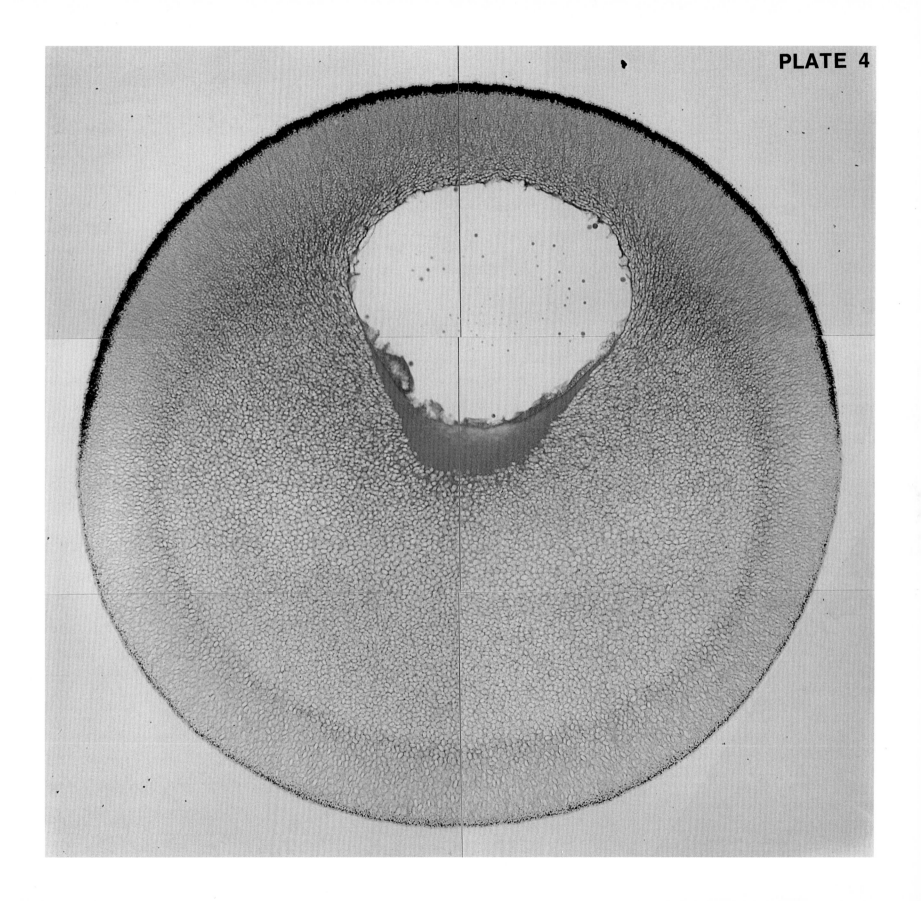

PLATE 4

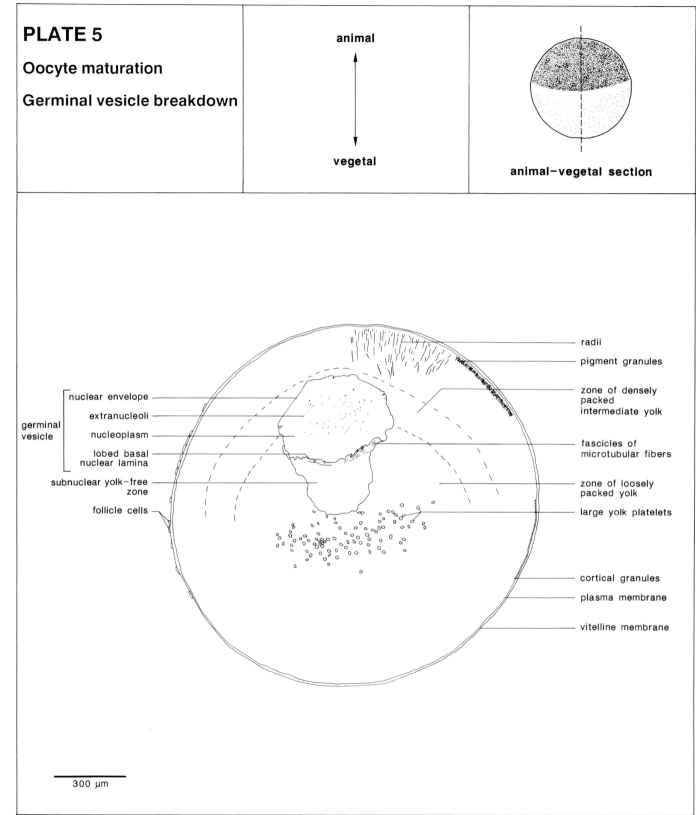

PLATE 5

Oocyte maturation

Germinal vesicle breakdown

animal

vegetal

animal–vegetal section

radii

pigment granules

zone of densely packed intermediate yolk

nuclear envelope

extranucleoli

germinal vesicle

nucleoplasm

lobed basal nuclear lamina

fascicles of microtubular fibers

subnuclear yolk-free zone

zone of loosely packed yolk

follicle cells

large yolk platelets

cortical granules

plasma membrane

vitelline membrane

300 μm

Progression of Germinal Vesicle Breakdown

Fascicles of microtubular fibers align tangentially to the basal side of the germinal vesicle (cf. PLATE 9D). The basal nuclear envelope shows signs of dissolution. Extranucleoli have become smaller. The subnuclear yolk-free zone extends further toward the center of the cell. This zone differs in structure and staining from the nucleoplasm, indicating that the subnuclear yolk-free zone and the nucleus still form two separate compartments. The packing of the yolk is loosened in the central region of the oocyte while intermediate yolk platelets appear in dense packing lateral to the germinal vesicle. (Staining: AAO)

PLATE 5

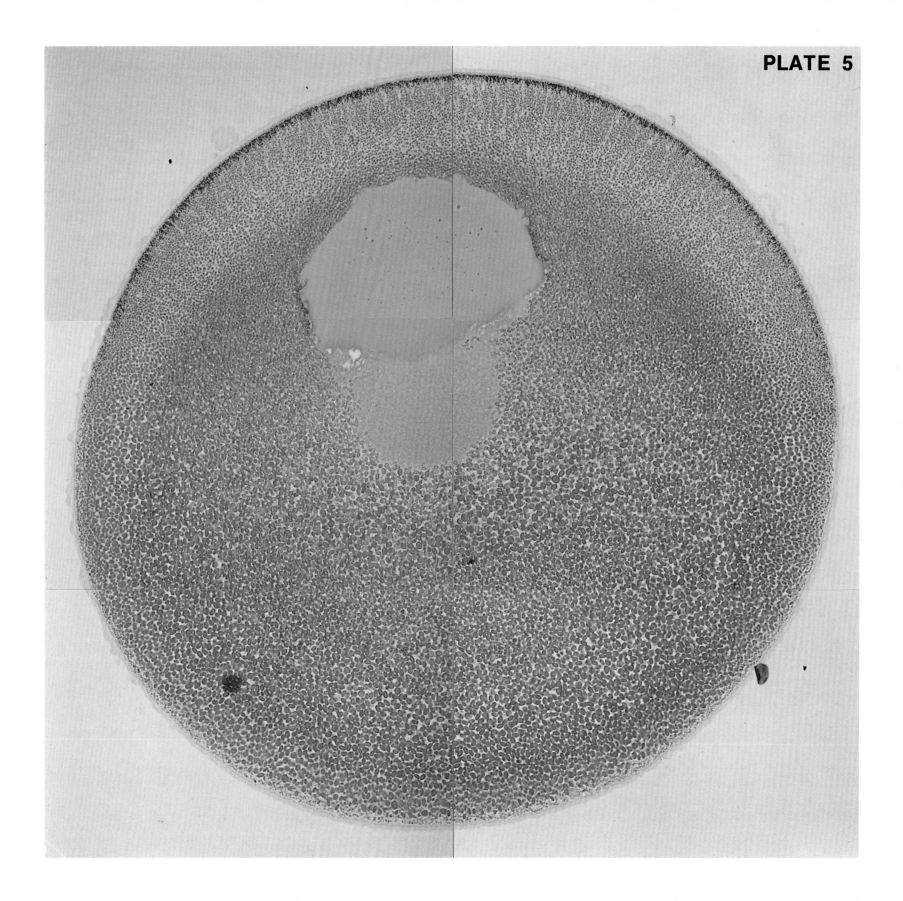

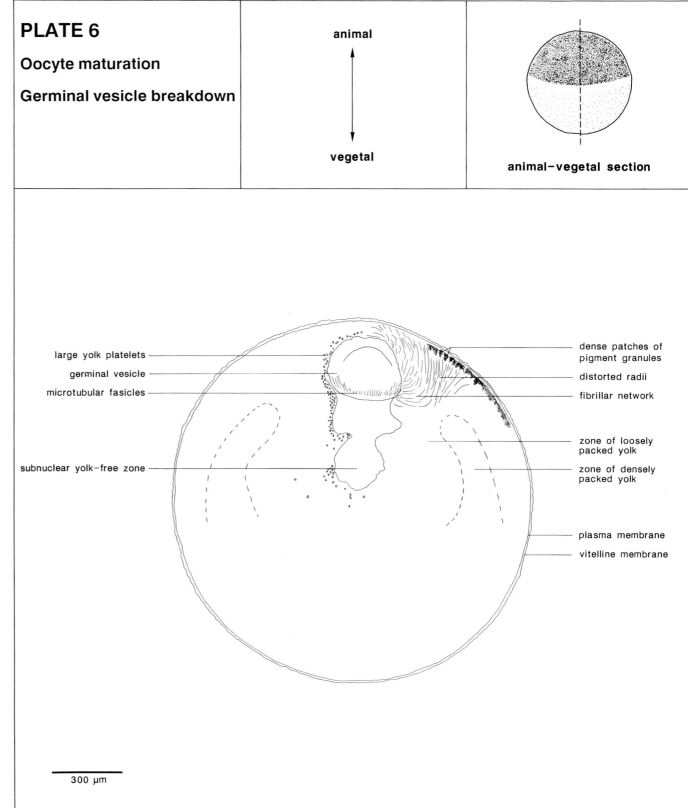

PLATE 6

Oocyte maturation

Germinal vesicle breakdown

animal

vegetal

animal–vegetal section

large yolk platelets

germinal vesicle

microtubular fasicles

subnuclear yolk-free zone

dense patches of
pigment granules

distorted radii

fibrillar network

zone of loosely
packed yolk

zone of densely
packed yolk

plasma membrane

vitelline membrane

300 µm

Progression of Germinal Vesicle Breakdown

The germinal vesicle has become smaller in size
and has moved toward the animal pole. Fascicles
of microtubuli invade the germinal vesicle from
its basal side (cf. PLATE 9E). Extranucleoli are
no longer visible. The subnuclear yolk-free zone
is large and extends to the center of the oocyte.
The system of the radii has become distorted.
Further cytoplasmic movements are indicated by
the displacement of yolk. The center of the oocyte seems to lose yolk, part of it being shifted laterally, while another part moves upwards along
the border of the yolk-free subnuclear zone. The
pigment of the animal cortex contracts into
patches and is slightly drawn inside. (Staining:
AAO)

PLATE 6

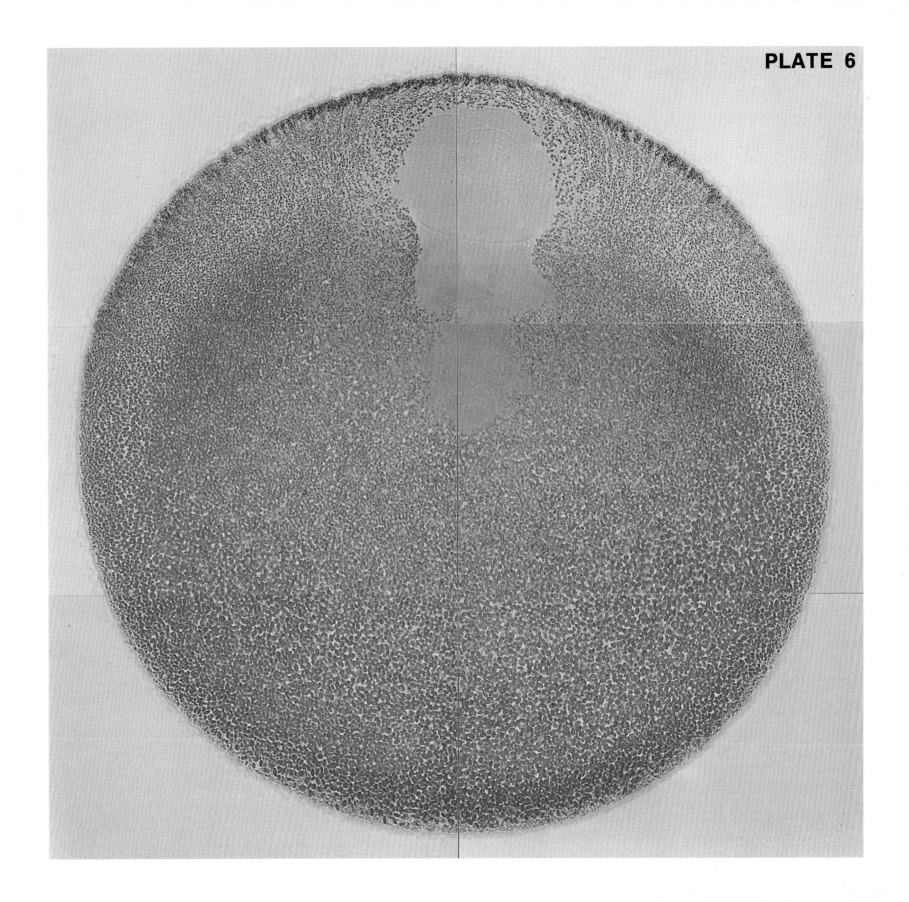

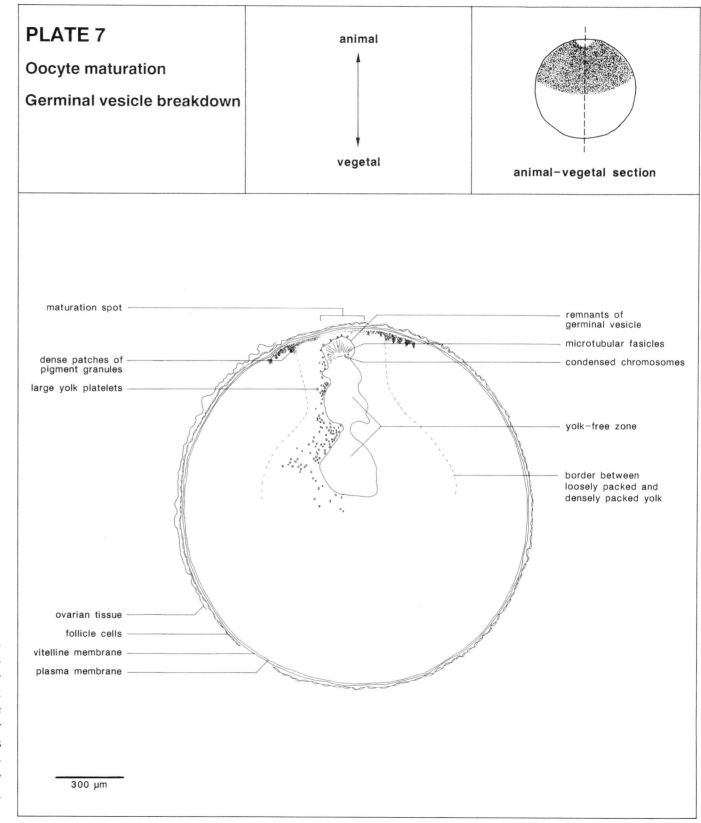

PLATE 7

Oocyte maturation

Germinal vesicle breakdown

animal

vegetal

animal–vegetal section

maturation spot

dense patches of
pigment granules

large yolk platelets

ovarian tissue

follicle cells

vitelline membrane

plasma membrane

remnants of
germinal vesicle

microtubular fasicles

condensed chromosomes

yolk-free zone

border between
loosely packed and
densely packed yolk

300 µm

Completion of Germinal Vesicle Breakdown

The germinal vesicle has almost disappeared, chromosomes are condensed and entangled in a network of microtubular fascicles, which is shifted toward the animal pole (cf. PLATE 9F). Yolk is displaced from the center of the cell, some large yolk platelets are collected along the border of the central yolk-free zone. The pigment has withdrawn from the animal pole, where the unpigmented maturation spot is forming. Laterally pigment patches have moved further inside. (Staining: AAO)

PLATE 7

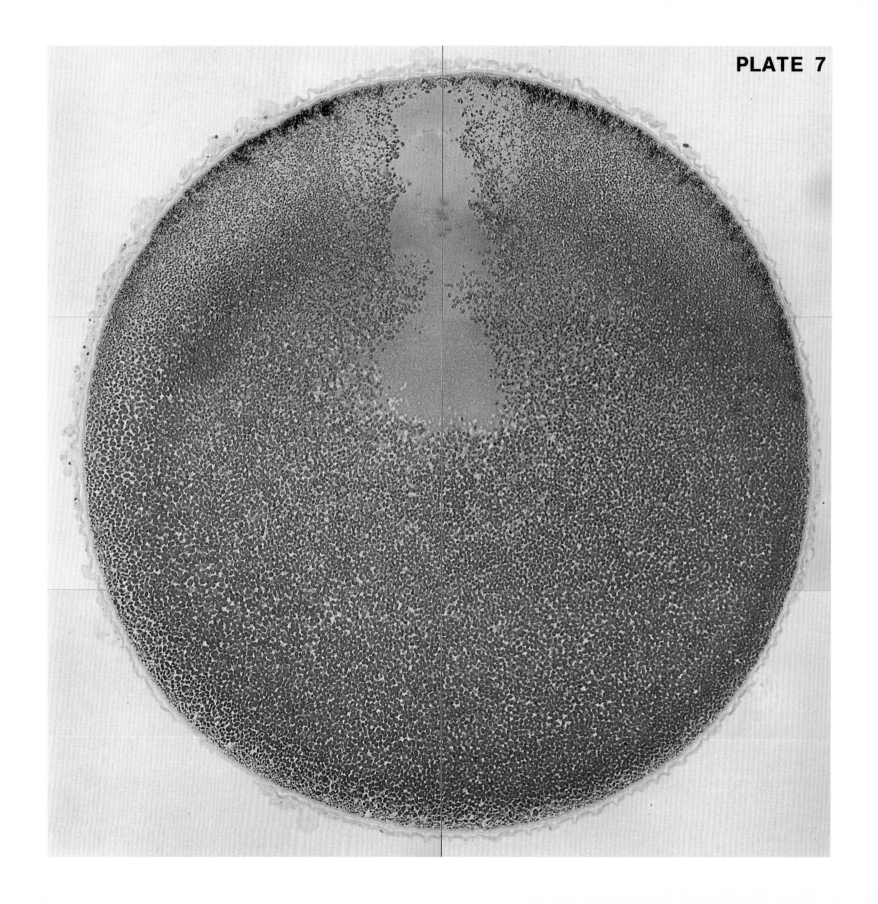

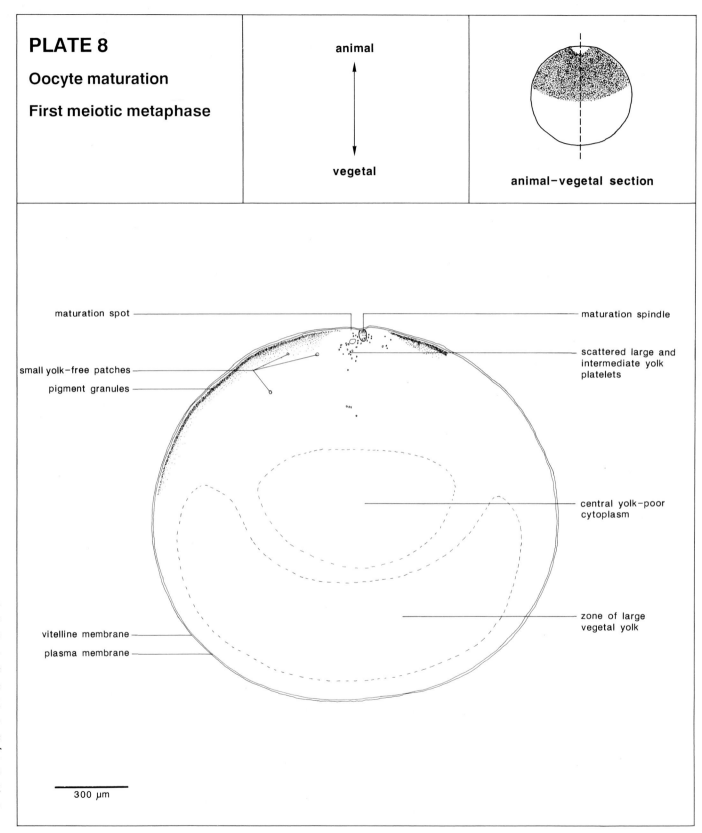

PLATE 8

Oocyte maturation

First meiotic metaphase

animal

vegetal

animal–vegetal section

maturation spot

maturation spindle

scattered large and intermediate yolk platelets

small yolk-free patches

pigment granules

central yolk-poor cytoplasm

zone of large vegetal yolk

vitelline membrane

plasma membrane

300 µm

Mature Egg

The condensed chromosomes are arranged in the maturation spindle, which is located in the center of the unpigmented maturation spot at the animal pole (cf. PLATE 9I). Most of the pigment has resumed its cortical position but some has remained in the subcortical cytoplasm. The center of the egg is occupied by yolk-poor and partially yolk-free cytoplasm. This region is obviously derived from the subnuclear yolk-free zone of the earlier stages. The vegetal region of the egg is not much affected by the cytoplasmic reorganization during maturation. Different eggs show a certain variation in their cytoplasmic organization. (Staining: AAO)

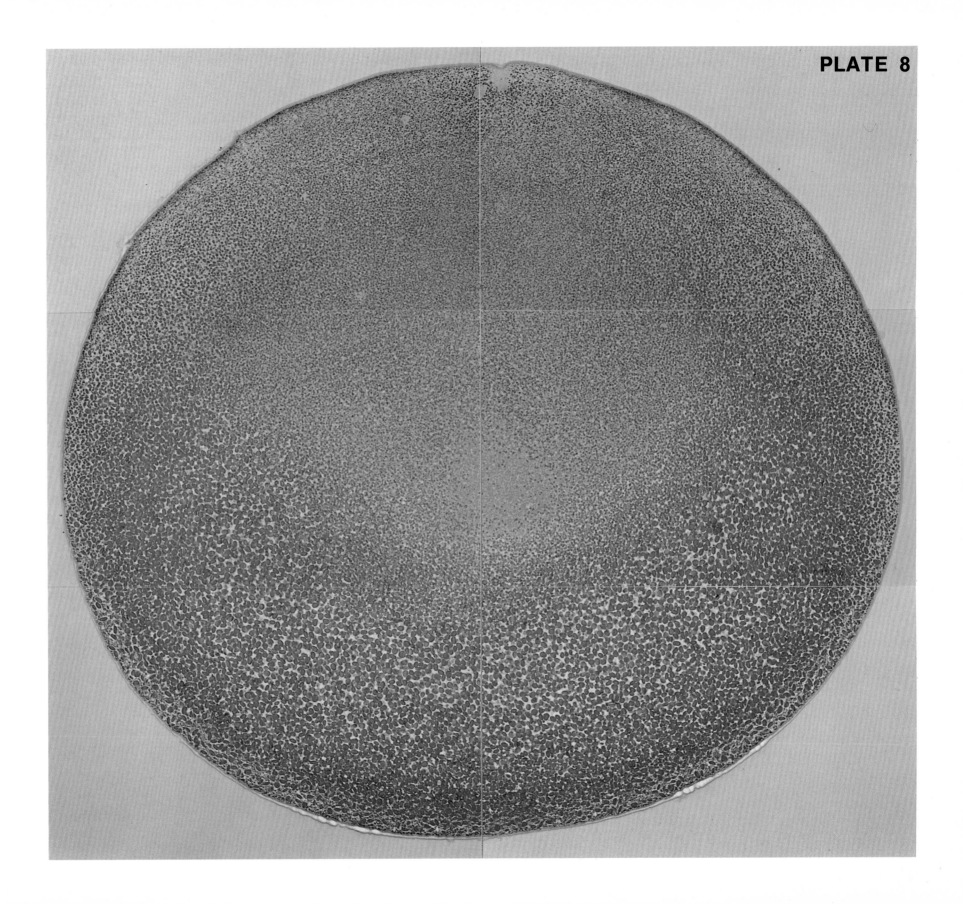

PLATE 8

PLATE 9

Oogenesis and Maturation

Nuclear Events during Meiosis at Higher Magnification

A Stage II Oocyte

Chromosomes with extended lampbrush loops are located in the center of the nucleus, the extranucleoli are located more in the periphery. (Staining: SFMB; magnification: 450x).

B Stage III Oocyte

The loops of the lampbrush chromosomes begin to retract. Nucleoli are more evenly scattered and heterogeneous in size. (Staining: AAO; magnification: 200x)

C Stage VI Oocyte

Nucleoli are different in size and more centrally located. (Staining: AAO; magnification: 200x)

D Oocyte Maturation

The onset of germinal vesicle breakdown is shown. Microtubular fascicles appear tangential to the basal nuclear membrane. (Staining: AAO; magnification: 200x)

E Oocyte Maturation

Microtubular fascicles invade the nucleus during germinal vesicle breakdown. Germinal vesicle breakdown has progressed to the stage depicted in PLATE 6. (Staining: AAO; magnification: 170x)

F Oocyte Maturation

Chromosomes are condensed and entangled in the microtubular system, which moves toward the oocyte periphery. Germinal vesicle breakdown has progressed to the stage depicted in PLATE 7. (Staining: AAO; magnification: 660x)

G Oocyte Maturation

Chromosomes are collected in the center of the microtubular system. (Staining: AAO; magnification: 850x)

H Oocyte Maturation

Chromosomes have reached the oocyte cortex at the animal pole. Note the pigment granules and the cortical granules, which are clearly visible at this magnification. (Staining: AAO; magnification: 850x)

I Completed Oocyte Maturation

The spindle of the first meiotic metaphase has formed. (Staining: AAO; magnification: 850x)

J, K Polar Body Extrusion

The formation of the second polar body is shown. Note that the cortical granules have disappeared due to exocytosis after fertilization. (Staining: AAO; magnification: 850x)

PLATE 9

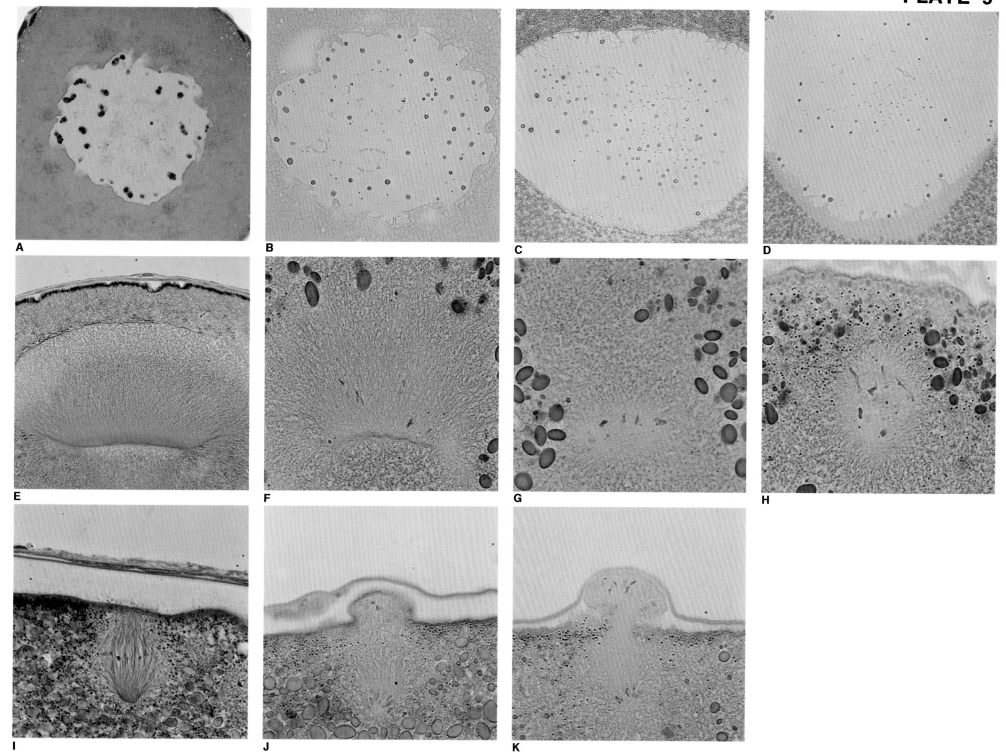

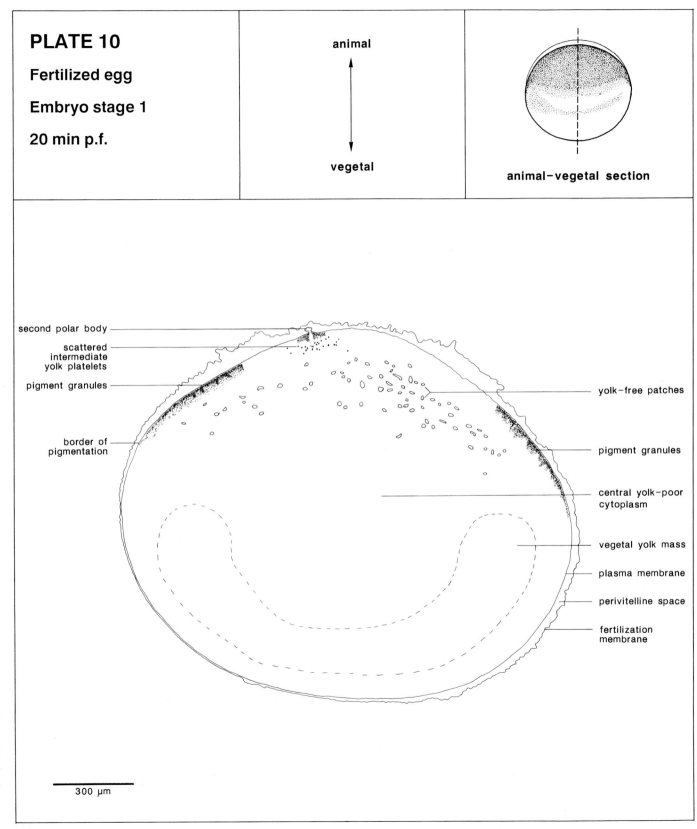

PLATE 10

Fertilized egg

Embryo stage 1

20 min p.f.

animal

↕

vegetal

animal−vegetal section

second polar body

scattered intermediate yolk platelets

pigment granules

border of pigmentation

yolk-free patches

pigment granules

central yolk-poor cytoplasm

vegetal yolk mass

plasma membrane

perivitelline space

fertilization membrane

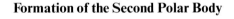

300 µm

Formation of the Second Polar Body

After fertilization the egg has performed the second meiotic division. The second polar body has been extruded. (The female pronucleus has formed, but is not visible in this section.) The animal cortex is contracted as indicated by the border of the animal pigment layer, which is lifted above the equator. The maturation spot has disappeared. Some of the pigment granules are found in the subcortical cytoplasm. A few intermediate yolk platelets, which represent a remnant of the maturation process, are located in the vicinity of the female pronucleus. The cortical granules have extruded their contents into the perivitelline space and have disappeared. The vitelline membrane has changed into the fertilization membrane and is lifted off the egg surface. (Staining: AAO)

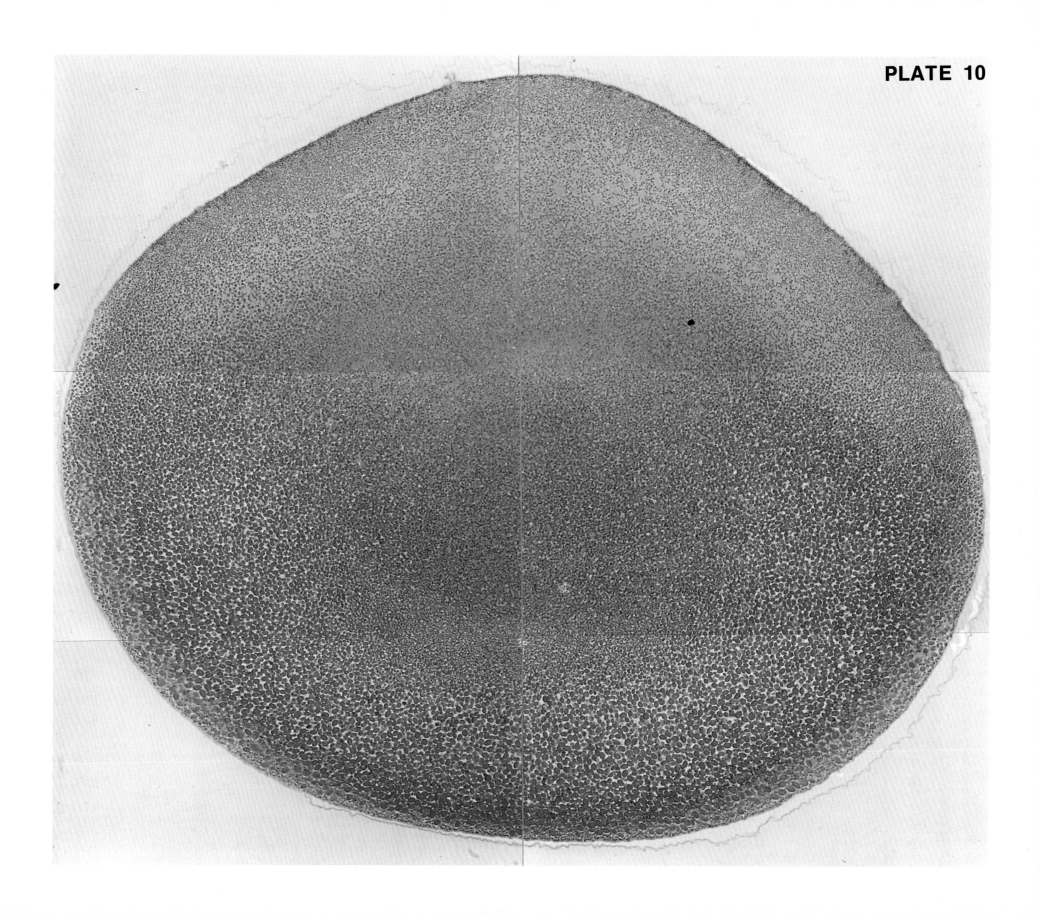

PLATE 10

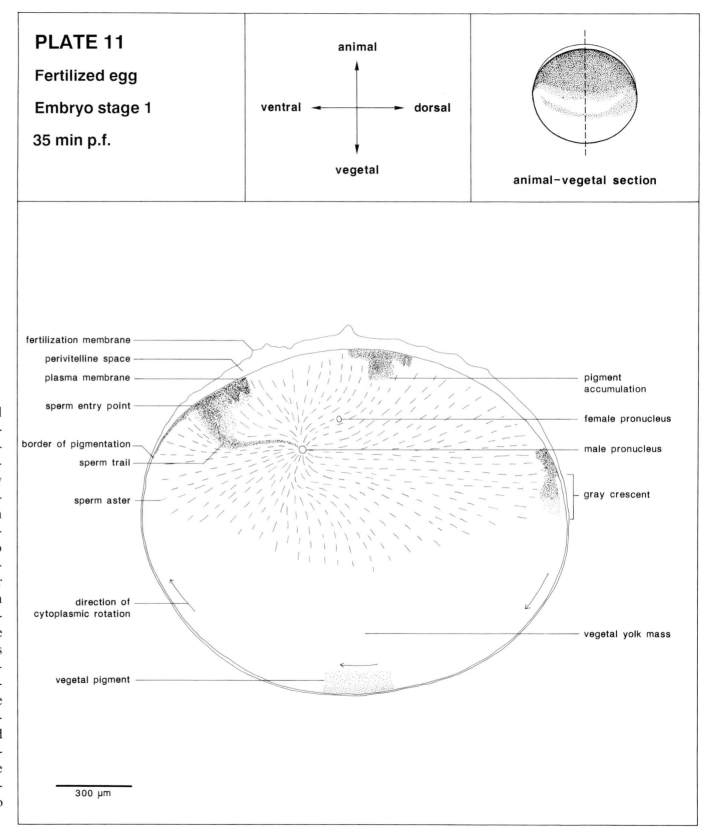

PLATE 11

Fertilized egg

Embryo stage 1

35 min p.f.

animal

ventral ← → dorsal

vegetal

animal–vegetal section

fertilization membrane
perivitelline space
plasma membrane

sperm entry point

border of pigmentation
sperm trail

sperm aster

direction of
cytoplasmic rotation

vegetal pigment

pigment
accumulation

female pronucleus

male pronucleus

gray crescent

vegetal yolk mass

300 µm

Pronuclear Migration

The sperm aster extends throughout the animal
hemisphere, the male pronucleus being the center of this microtubular system. Some of the pigment has moved from the cortex into the underlying cytoplasm. The sperm trail is marked by
pigment containing cortical material. A conspicuous accumulation of pigment marks the sperm
entry point at the future ventral side. The original position of the female pronucleus is also
marked by a pigment accumulation. The pigment arrangement at the animal-vegetal border
is indicative of the rotation of the cytoplasm
within the cortical shell: the pigment of the cortex remains in its original position, whereas the
pigment that has invaded the cytoplasm takes
part in the rotation. In this way unpigmented vegetal cytoplasm comes to lie underneath the pigmented animal cortex on the ventral side of the
egg and dorsally the pigmented animal cytoplasm comes to lie underneath the unpigmented
vegetal cortex. This latter configuration constitutes the gray crescent. The curved shape of the
sperm trail may also be a result of this cytoplasmic movement. Pigment ingression has also
occurred at the vegetal side. (Staining: azure B)

PLATE 11

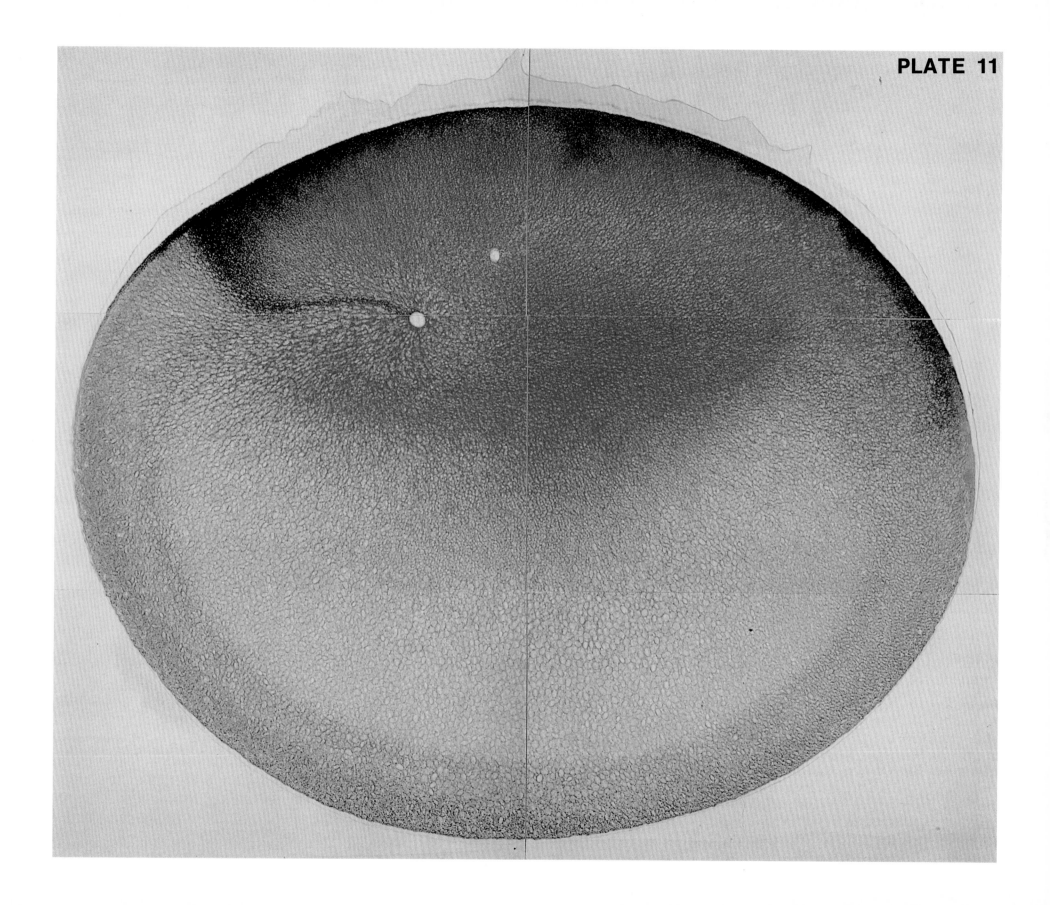

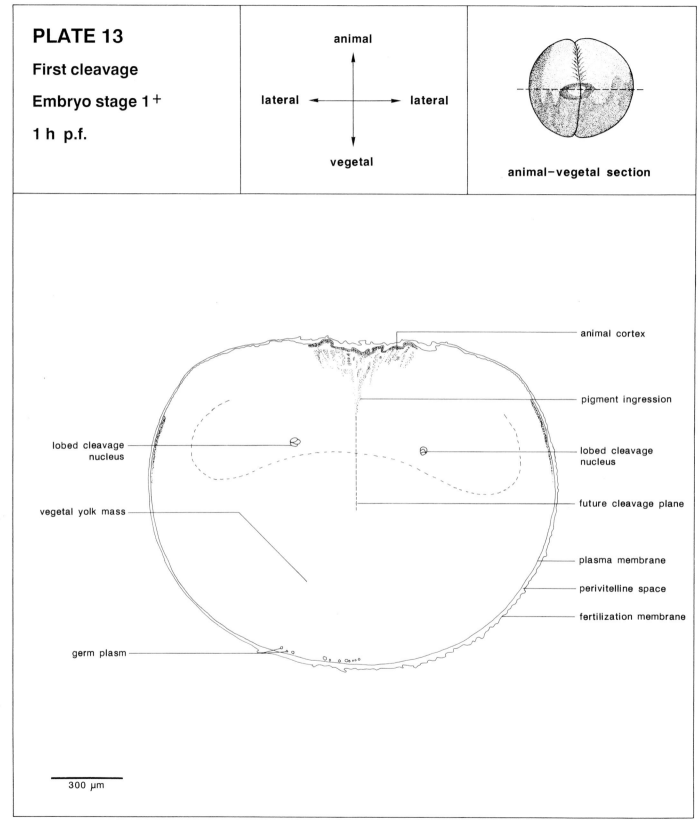

PLATE 13

First cleavage

Embryo stage 1⁺

1 h p.f.

animal

lateral ← → lateral

vegetal

animal–vegetal section

animal cortex

pigment ingression

lobed cleavage nucleus

lobed cleavage nucleus

future cleavage plane

vegetal yolk mass

plasma membrane

perivitelline space

fertilization membrane

germ plasm

300 µm

Telophase of First Cleavage Division, Onset of Cytokinesis

The animal cortex is wrinkled and contracted, the cytoplasmic pigment is aggregated in patches. Some pigment has moved to the interior along the future cleavage plane (indicating cortical ingression). The future cleavage plane is also foreshadowed by the arrangement of yolk in the animal cytoplasm. The two cleavage nuclei exhibit the typical lobed appearance. Laterally, the pigment has returned to the cortex. Patches of germ plasm begin to appear near the vegetal cortex. The cytoplasm is more clearly segregated into an animal and a vegetal domain than in earlier stages. Note the precise symmetry of cytoplasmic arrangement in the two halves of the animal hemisphere. (Staining: AAO)

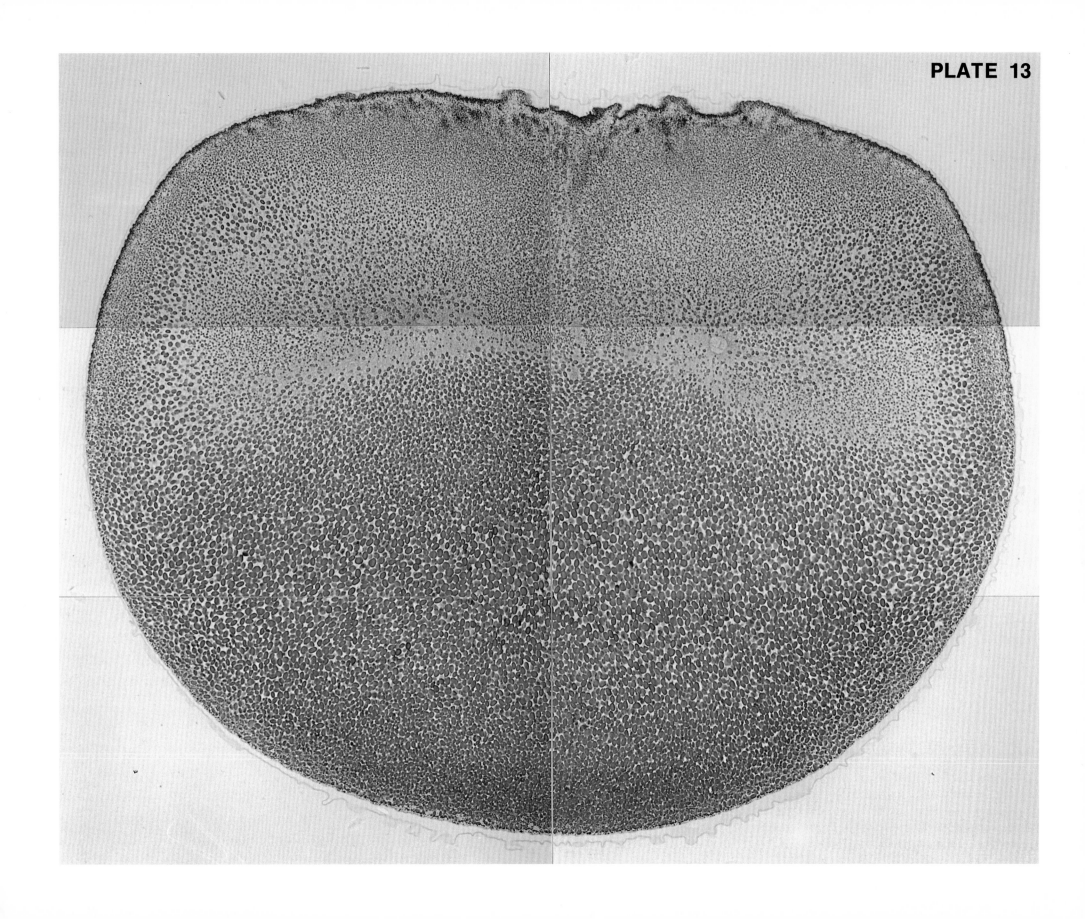

PLATE 13

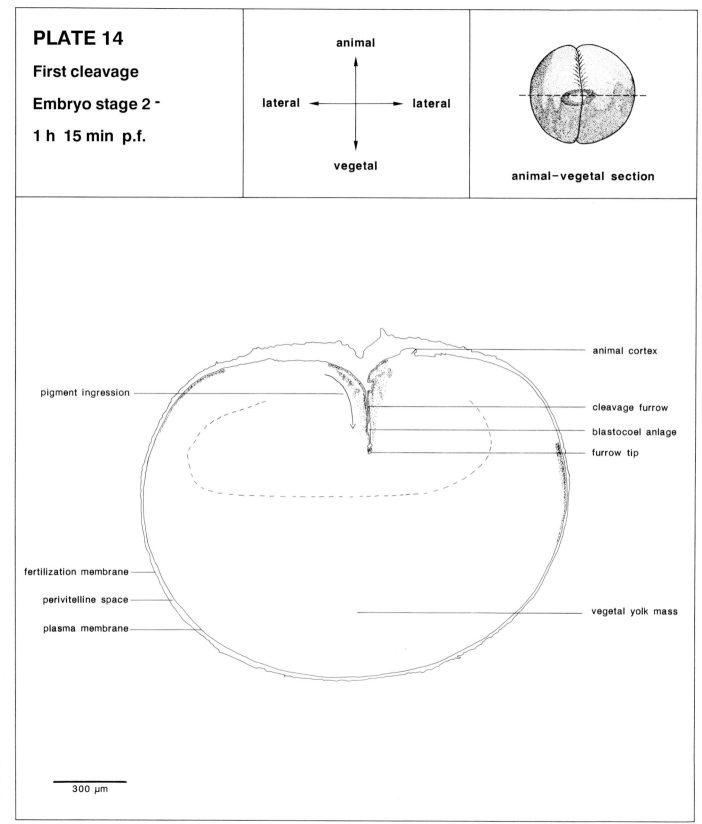

PLATE 14

First cleavage

Embryo stage 2 -

1 h 15 min p.f.

animal

lateral ← → lateral

vegetal

animal–vegetal section

animal cortex

pigment ingression

cleavage furrow

blastocoel anlage

furrow tip

fertilization membrane

perivitelline space

plasma membrane

vegetal yolk mass

300 μm

Early First Cleavage

The animal plasma membrane and the underlying cortex are drawn into the cleavage furrow. The larger vesicle in the furrow represents the blastocoel anlage. The vesicles at the furrow tip are the preferential sites of new membrane formation. (Staining: AAO)

PLATE 14

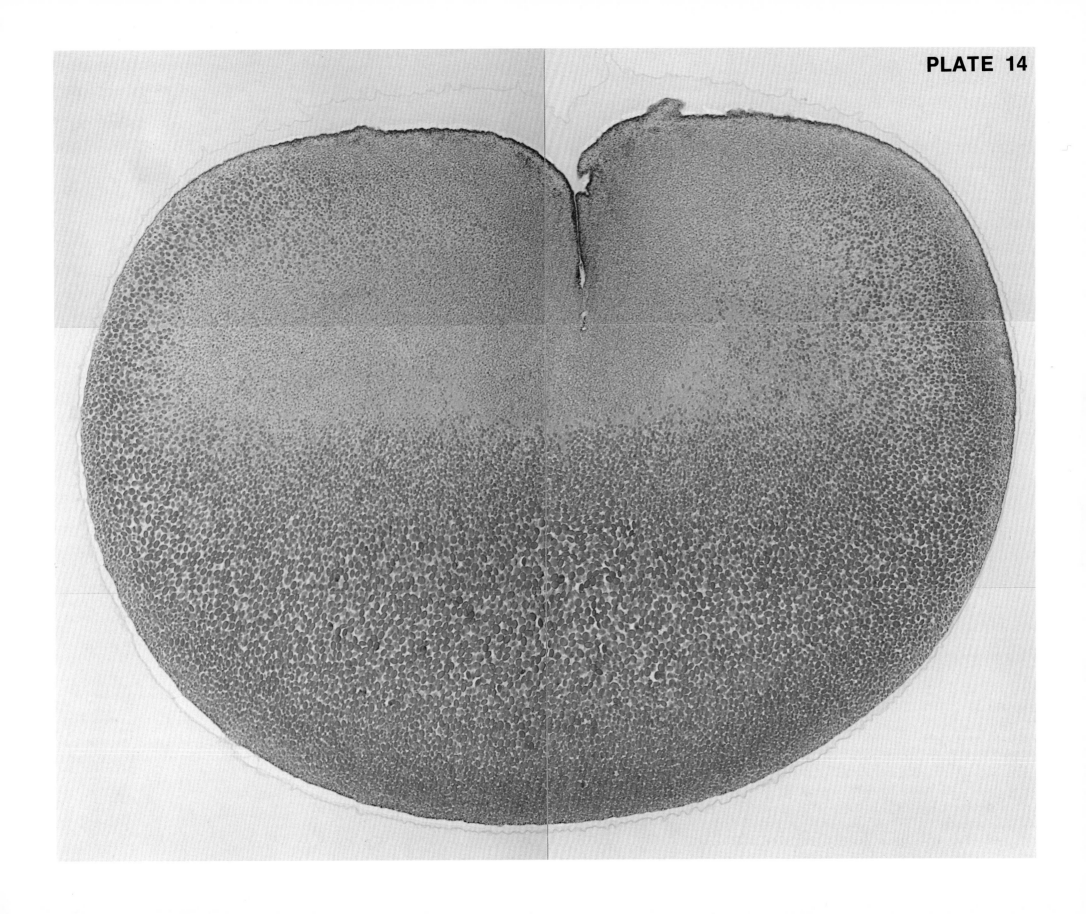

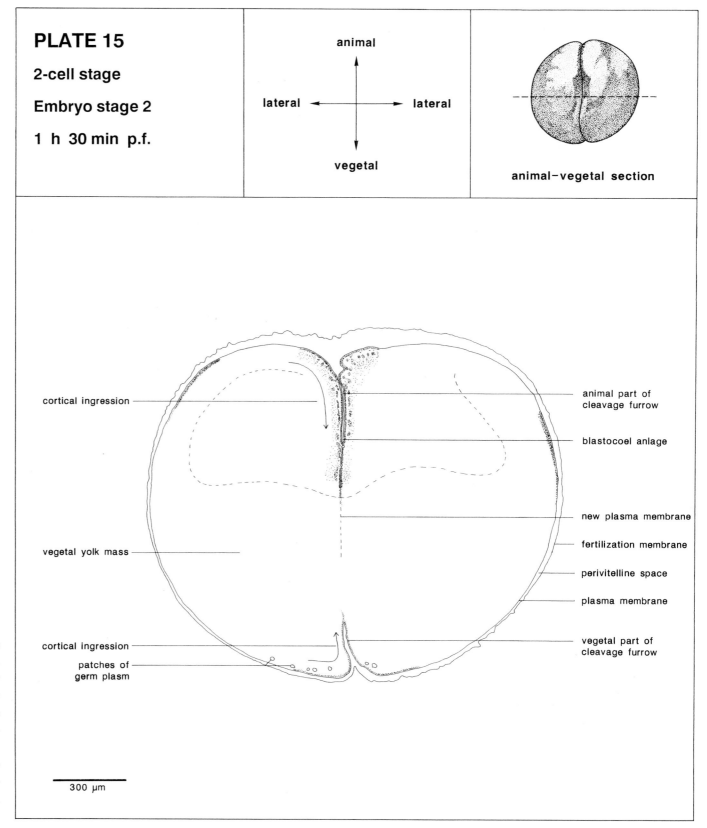

PLATE 15

2-cell stage

Embryo stage 2

1 h 30 min p.f.

animal

lateral ← → lateral

vegetal

animal–vegetal section

cortical ingression

animal part of
cleavage furrow

blastocoel anlage

new plasma membrane

fertilization membrane

perivitelline space

plasma membrane

vegetal yolk mass

vegetal part of
cleavage furrow

cortical ingression

patches of
germ plasm

300 µm

Completion of the First Cleavage Division

Pigment has moved along the cleavage plane deep into the center of the egg, indicating the ingression of cortical material which was originally localized beneath the membrane of the egg. The animal-vegetal asymmetry of the cleavage process has led to the formation of a deep animal furrow with vesicles and a shallow vegetal furrow. The newly formed membrane connecting the animal and vegetal furrows is not visible. The aggregation of germ plasm near the vegetal cortex has continued. (Staining: AAO)

PLATE 15

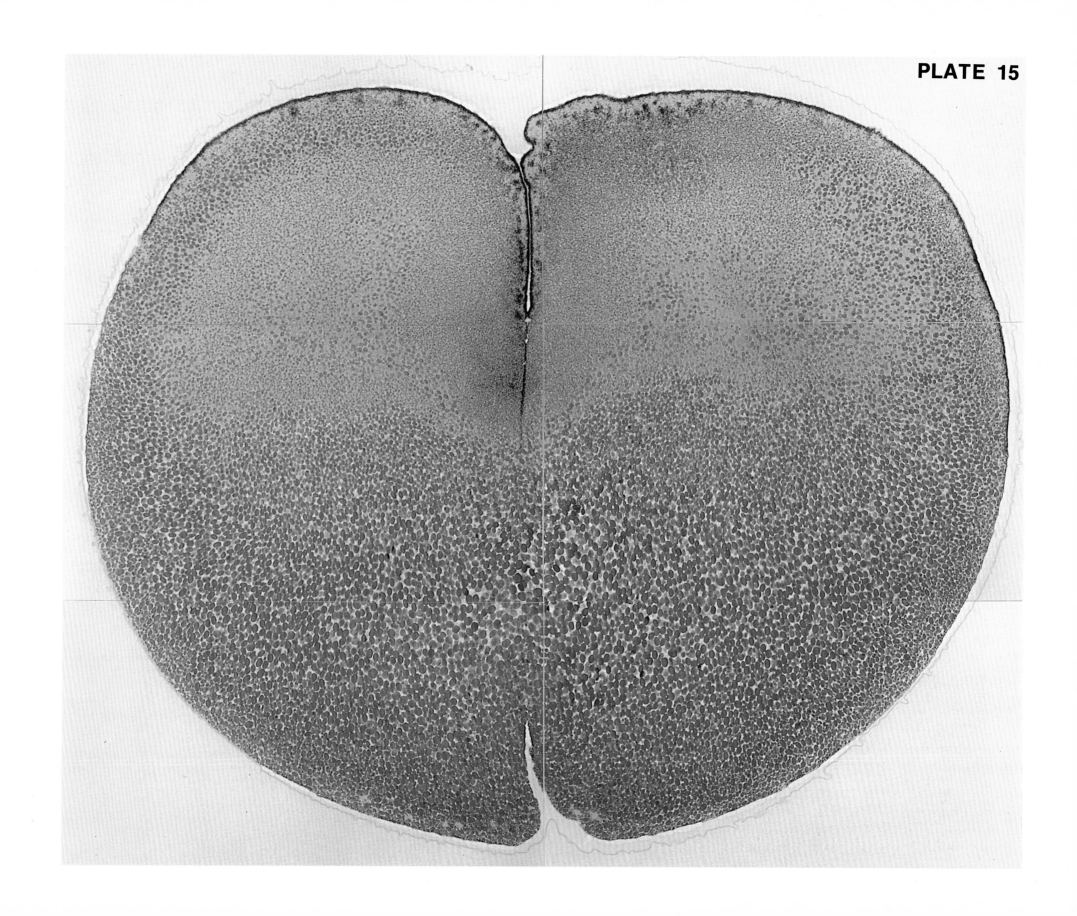

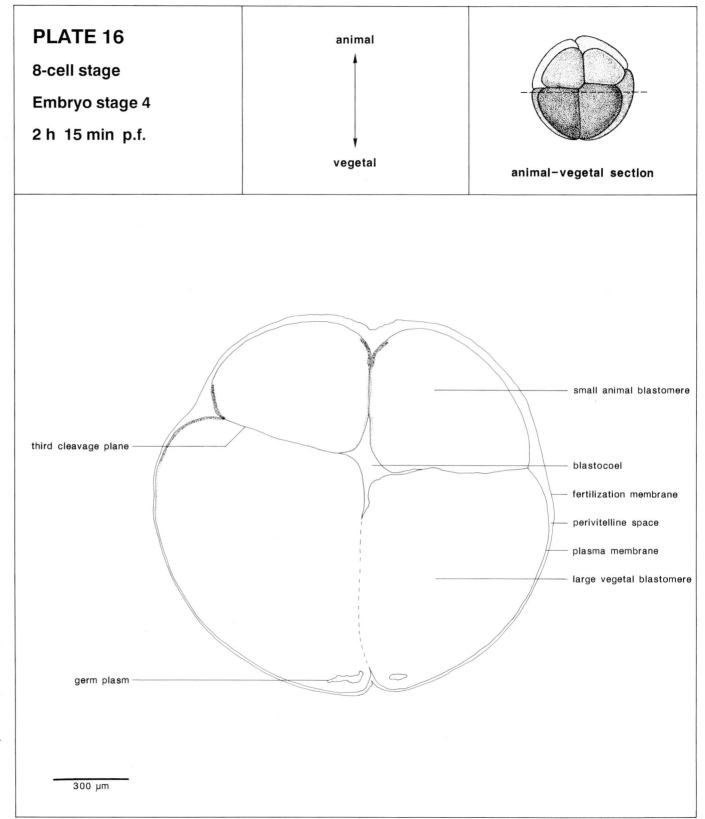

PLATE 16

8-cell stage

Embryo stage 4

2 h 15 min p.f.

animal

vegetal

animal–vegetal section

small animal blastomere

third cleavage plane

blastocoel

fertilization membrane

perivitelline space

plasma membrane

large vegetal blastomere

germ plasm

300 µm

Completion of the Third Cleavage Division

The animal and vegetal compartments of the egg are separated by the third cleavage plane. The difference in size and in cytoplasmic contents between the animal and vegetal blastomeres is obvious. Apically the cells are connected by close junctions, which seal off the blastocoel cavity from the surrounding medium. The germ plasm is fully aggregated. In the further process of cleavage, the germ plasm will be shifted toward the interior of the vegetal blastomeres as a result of continuing cortical ingression. (Staining: AAO)

PLATE 16

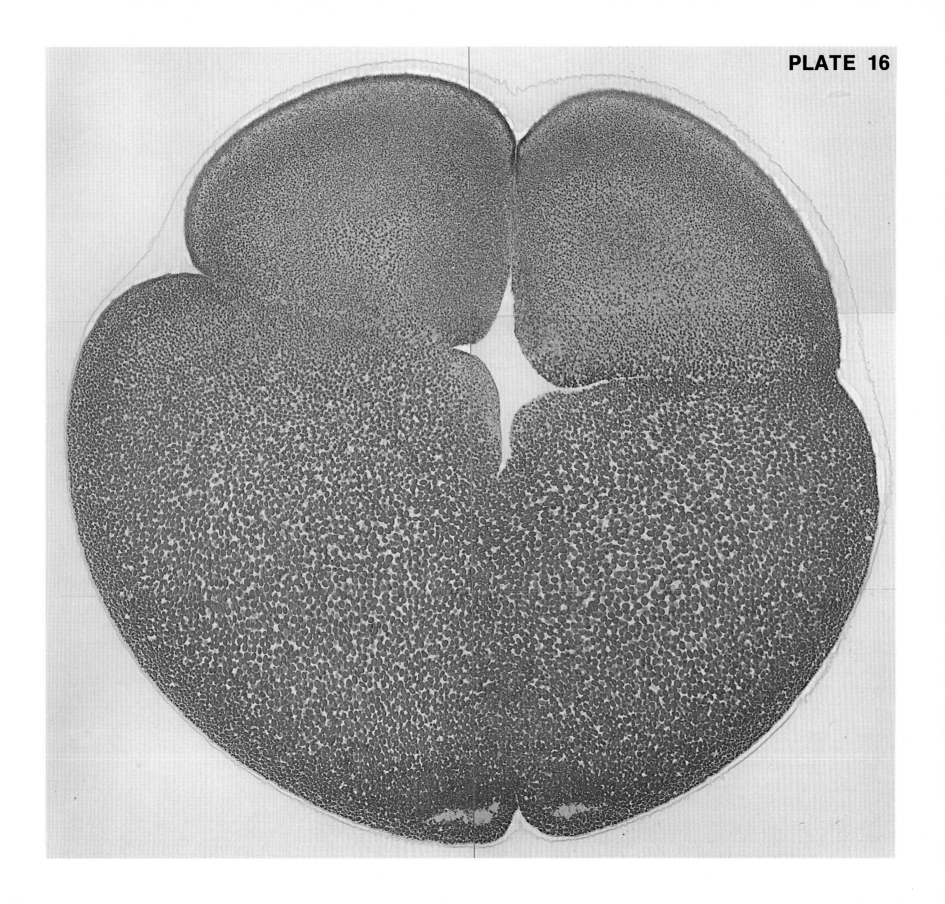

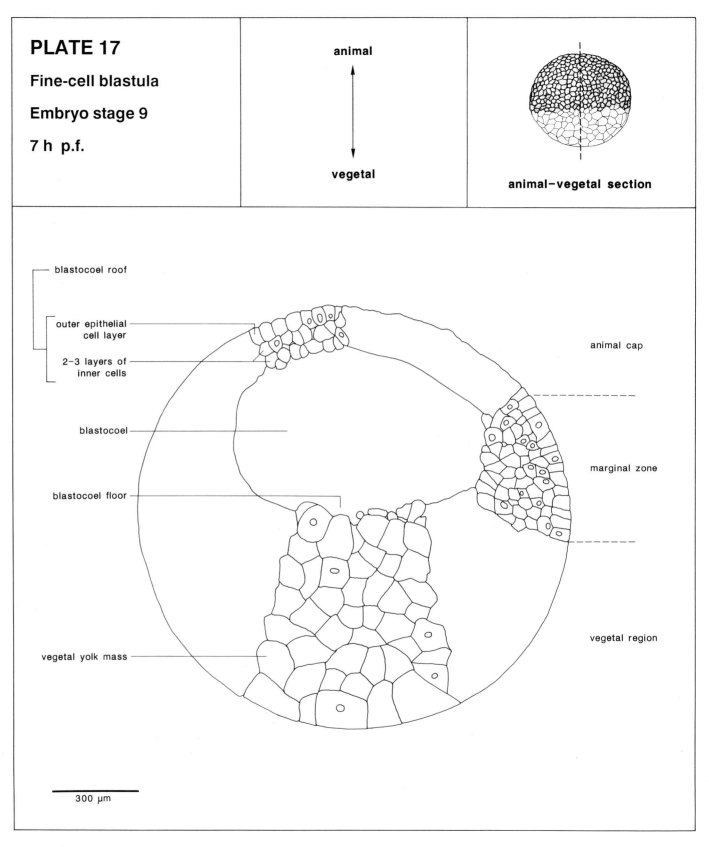

PLATE 17

Fine-cell blastula

Embryo stage 9

7 h p.f.

animal

vegetal

animal–vegetal section

blastocoel roof

outer epithelial
cell layer

2–3 layers of
inner cells

blastocoel

blastocoel floor

vegetal yolk mass

animal cap

marginal zone

vegetal region

300 μm

Late Midblastula

The blastocoel is large and contains a coarse precipitate of the blastocoel contents. The blastocoel roof consists of three to four cell layers. Animal and vegetal cells differ in size and arrangement. In the vegetal region the cell shape is adapted to maximal cell contact, in the animal region the cells appear more rounded leaving spaces between the cells. In the vegetal region the outer surface of the epithelial cell layer is smoother and straighter than in the animal cap region. Animal cells begin to be shifted below the equator, indicating the onset of the pregastrula epibolic movement. (Staining: BCB)

PLATE 17

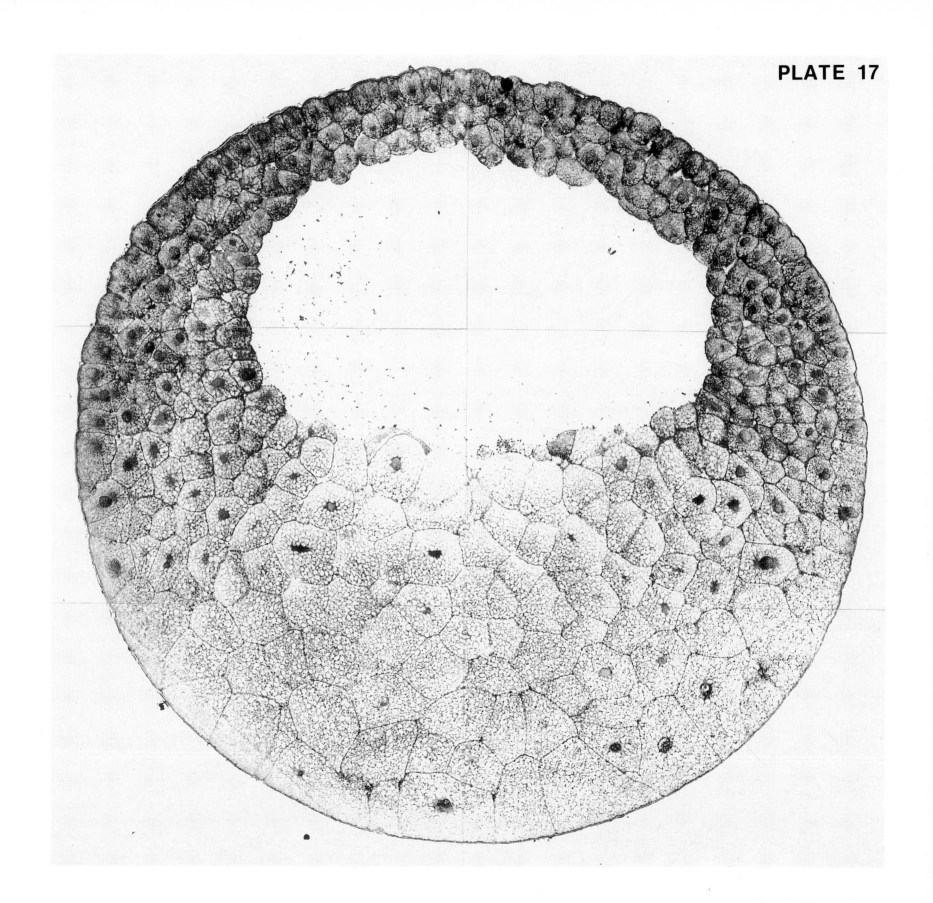

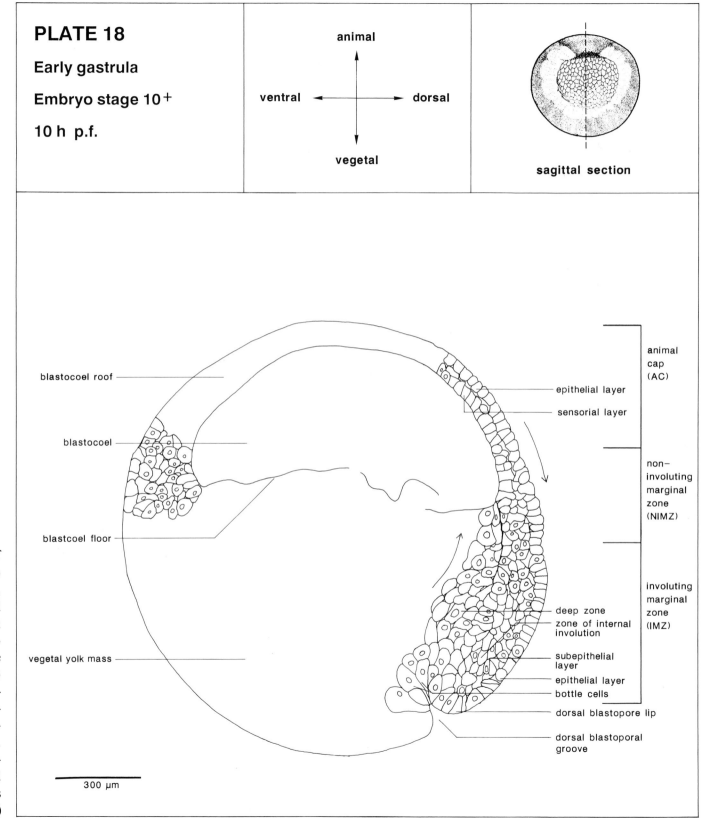

PLATE 18

Early gastrula

Embryo stage 10+

10 h p.f.

animal

ventral ← → dorsal

vegetal

sagittal section

blastocoel roof

blastocoel

blastcoel floor

vegetal yolk mass

300 µm

epithelial layer

sensorial layer

animal cap (AC)

non-involuting marginal zone (NIMZ)

involuting marginal zone (IMZ)

deep zone

zone of internal involution

subepithelial layer

epithelial layer

bottle cells

dorsal blastopore lip

dorsal blastoporal groove

Onset of Gastrulation

Radial intercalation has led to a thinning out of the blastocoel roof, which now consists of two layers: the outer, epithelial layer and the inner, sensorial layer. The expansion of the blastocoel roof by epibolic movement is more advanced on the dorsal side, where animal material is constantly shifted vegetally (*arrow*). Bottle cells have formed at the blastopore and have begun to move inwards. The subepithelial suprablastoporal cells involute internally and move animalwards. The cells of the deep zone move animalwards, approaching the blastocoel roof (*arrow*). These processes have not yet begun on the ventral side. The boundary between NIMZ and IMZ is not easy to locate; the drawing indicates this border only approximately. (Staining: BCB)

PLATE 18

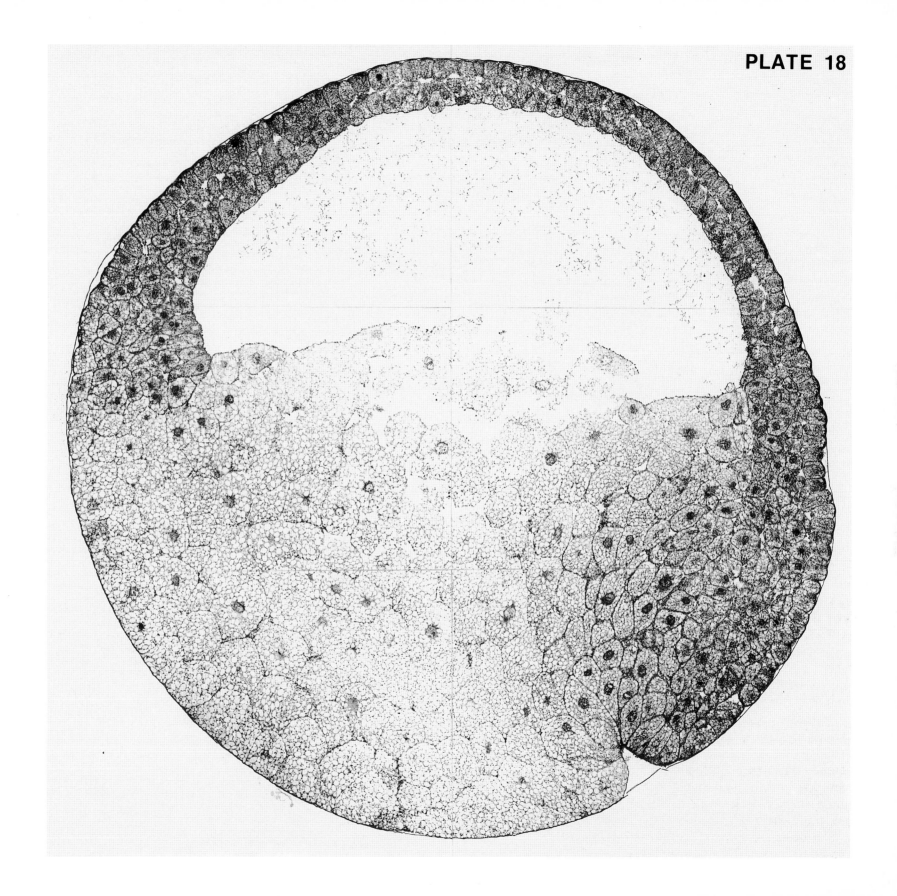

PLATE 19

Large yolk plug stage

Embryo stage 11 1/2

12 h 15 min p.f.

animal

dorsal ← → ventral

vegetal

sagittal section

Midgastrula

Involution on the dorsal side has advanced. The bottle cells have moved into the interior, marking the tip of the slit-shaped archenteron. The epithelium forming the archenteron roof represents the involuted, superficial, suprablastoporal epithelium. The dorsal suprablastoporal region contains a massive accumulation of cells which have been shifted dorsally from the lateral regions by dorsal convergence and animalwards by extension. The axial mesoderm begins to form from these cells. Cell arrangement within the dorsal blastopore lip appears chaotic, an ordered involution around an inner lip cannot be discerned. The vegetal yolk mass is "overrolled" by the advancing dorsal blastopore lip. Spreading mesodermal cells from the deep zone and adjacent endodermal cells from the vegetal yolk mass are approaching the animal pole. Larger and further advanced mesodermal cells are not easily distinguished from endodermal cells. The three germ layers begin to become discernible. As a first sign of neural induction the cells of the sensorial layer of the dorsal ectoderm (prospective neurectoderm) begin to elongate and form a columnar epithelium. Contrary to current theories on neural induction, this happens also at the animal pole, which is not in contact with mesodermal cells. Bottle cell formation has reached the ventral side, where the number of prospective mesodermal cells migrating in the animal direction is smaller than on the dorsal side. The depression at the blastocoel roof is an artifact resulting from the embedding procedure. (Staining: BCB)

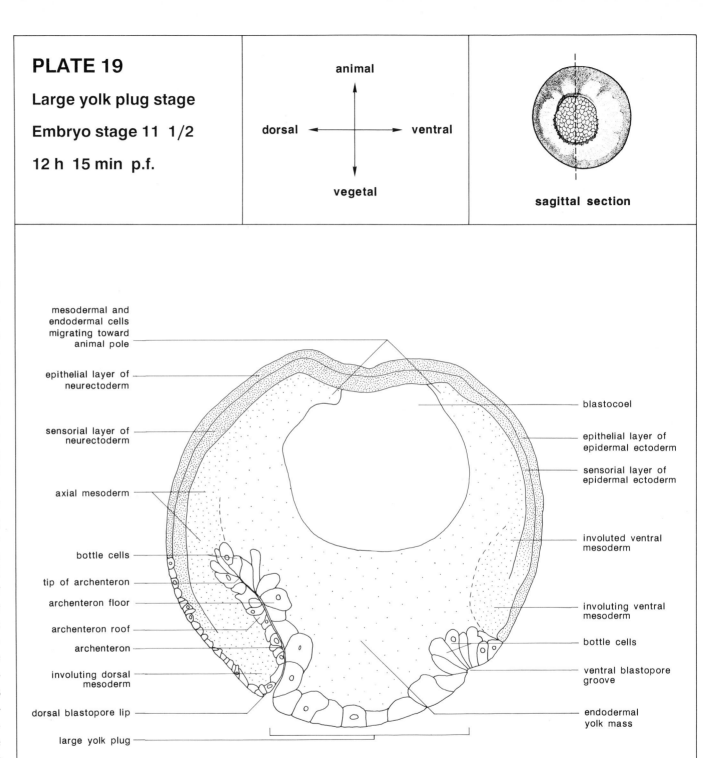

mesodermal and endodermal cells migrating toward animal pole

epithelial layer of neurectoderm

sensorial layer of neurectoderm

axial mesoderm

bottle cells

tip of archenteron

archenteron floor

archenteron roof

archenteron

involuting dorsal mesoderm

dorsal blastopore lip

large yolk plug

blastocoel

epithelial layer of epidermal ectoderm

sensorial layer of epidermal ectoderm

involuted ventral mesoderm

involuting ventral mesoderm

bottle cells

ventral blastopore groove

endodermal yolk mass

300 µm

PLATE 19

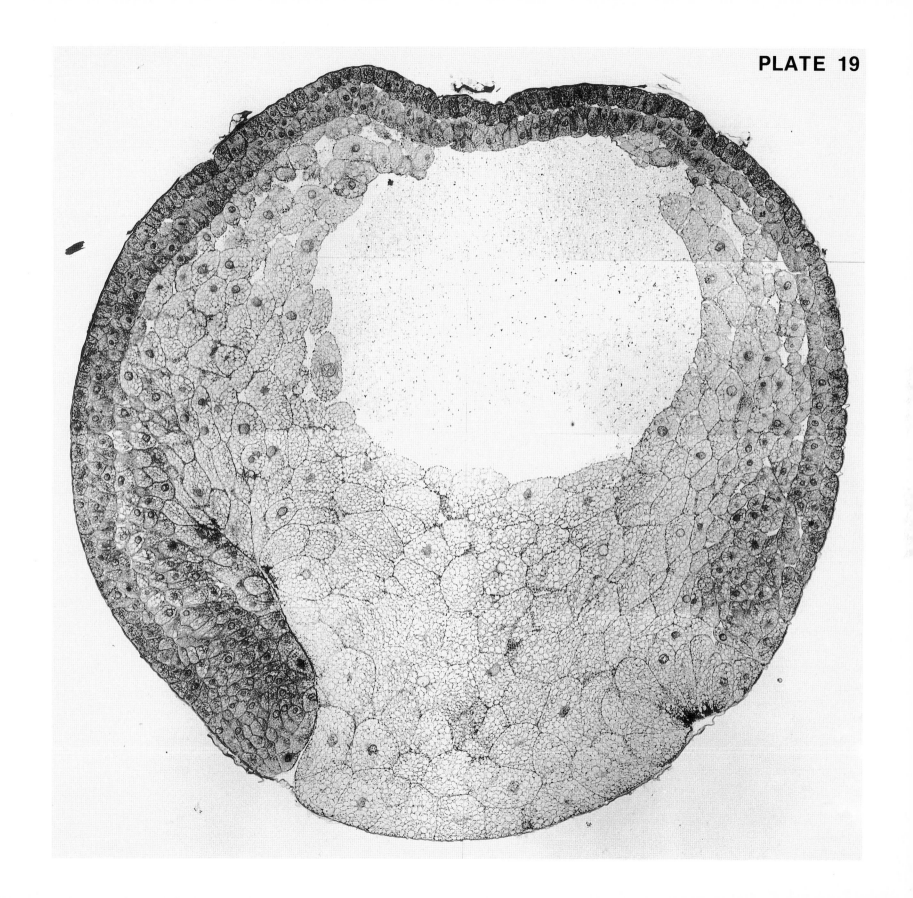

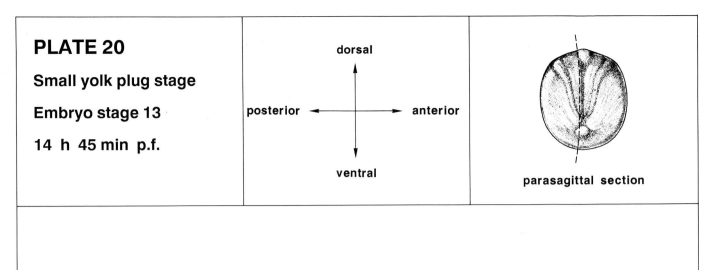

PLATE 20

Small yolk plug stage

Embryo stage 13

14 h 45 min p.f.

dorsal

posterior ← → anterior

ventral

parasagittal section

Advanced Gastrula

The archenteron has become inflated at the expense of the blastocoel, which is markedly displaced ventrally. The archenteron roof is formed by involuted, superficial cells of the suprablastoporal region. Bottle cells have respread and contribute to the lining of the archenteron. The archenteron floor consists of cells derived from the outer epithelial lining of the vegetal yolk mass. The arrangement of the mesodermal cells at the site of involution appears to be disordered (but cf. PLATE 22 A). More to the anterior the cells of the paraxial mesoderm align in dorsoventral direction. The anterior region of the mesodermal layer is occupied by the spreading prechordal plate cells. They are not easy to discern from the cells of the head endoderm. The induction of the neural plate has resulted in a columnarization of the cells of the sensorial layer of the induced dorsal ectoderm (neurectoderm).

Involution on the ventral side is less advanced. Bottle cells are drawn to the inside but have not yet spread. The amount of mesodermal material at the ventral site of involution is small compared to that on the dorsal side. Spreading mesodermal cells have reached the original animal pole. They always keep close contact with the adjacent endodermal cells. The blastopore has normally closed to a narrow slit at this stage. In this specimen it has remained unusually large. This variability is often encountered in *Xenopus* development; it does not affect the normal progression of embryogenesis. (Staining: BCB)

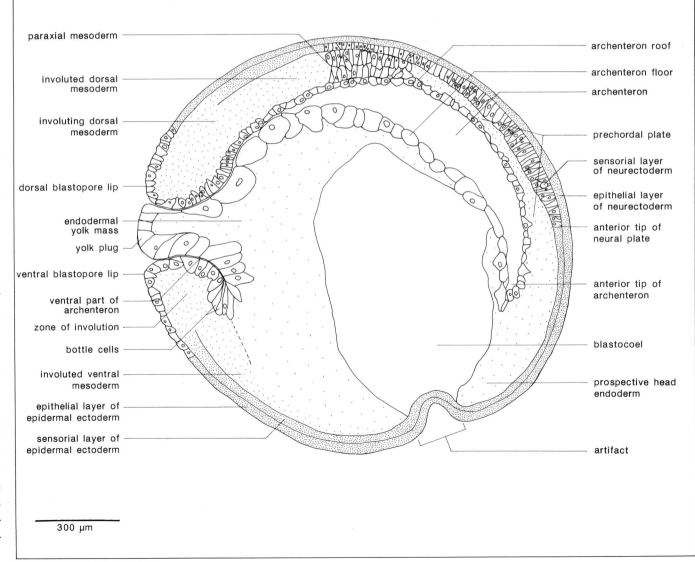

paraxial mesoderm

involuted dorsal mesoderm

involuting dorsal mesoderm

dorsal blastopore lip

endodermal yolk mass

yolk plug

ventral blastopore lip

ventral part of archenteron

zone of involution

bottle cells

involuted ventral mesoderm

epithelial layer of epidermal ectoderm

sensorial layer of epidermal ectoderm

archenteron roof

archenteron floor

archenteron

prechordal plate

sensorial layer of neurectoderm

epithelial layer of neurectoderm

anterior tip of neural plate

anterior tip of archenteron

blastocoel

prospective head endoderm

artifact

300 µm

PLATE 20

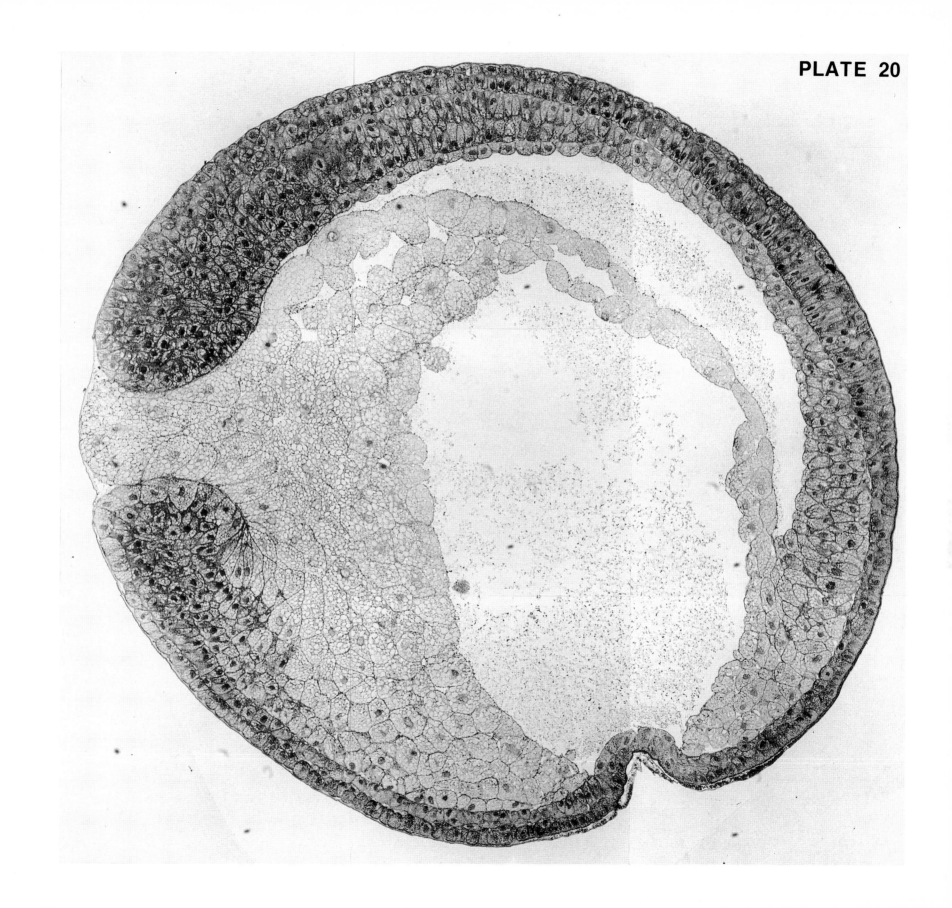

PLATE 21

Small yolk plug stage

Embryo stage 12 1/2

14 h 30 min p.f.

dorsal

↕

ventral

central transversal section

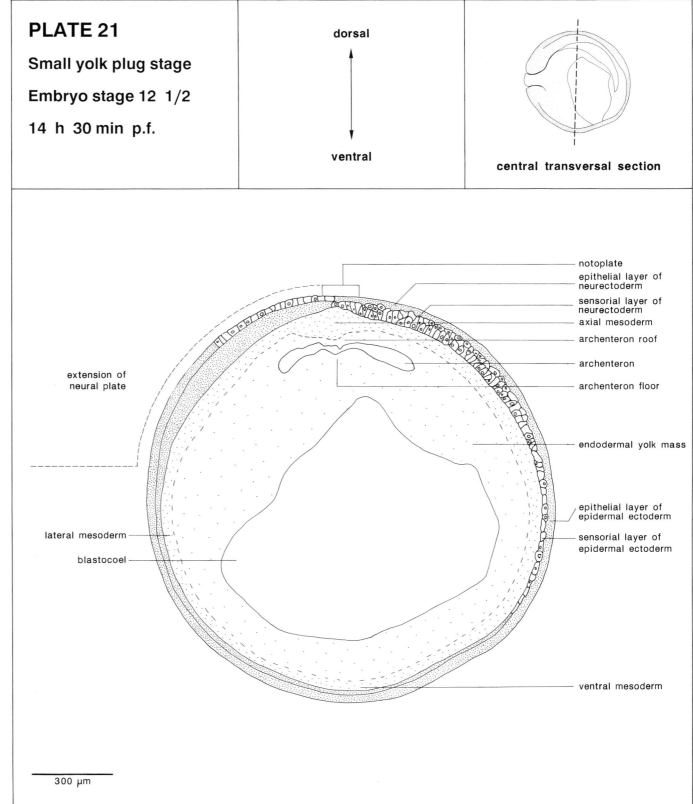

notoplate

epithelial layer of neurectoderm

sensorial layer of neurectoderm

axial mesoderm

archenteron roof

archenteron

archenteron floor

endodermal yolk mass

epithelial layer of epidermal ectoderm

sensorial layer of epidermal ectoderm

ventral mesoderm

extension of neural plate

lateral mesoderm

blastocoel

300 μm

Advanced Gastrula

The neural plate is indicated by the columnarization of the sensorial layer of the neurectoderm. The dorsal midline of the neural plate is occupied by the notoplate, in which the cells of both ectodermal layers are markedly thinner. There is no sharp boundary between neurectoderm and the lateral epidermal ectoderm. The section passes through the anterior tip of the axial mesoderm where the notochord is only vaguely delimited. The lateral and ventral mesoderm is distinguished from the endodermal yolk mass by the difference in cell size. (Staining: BCB)

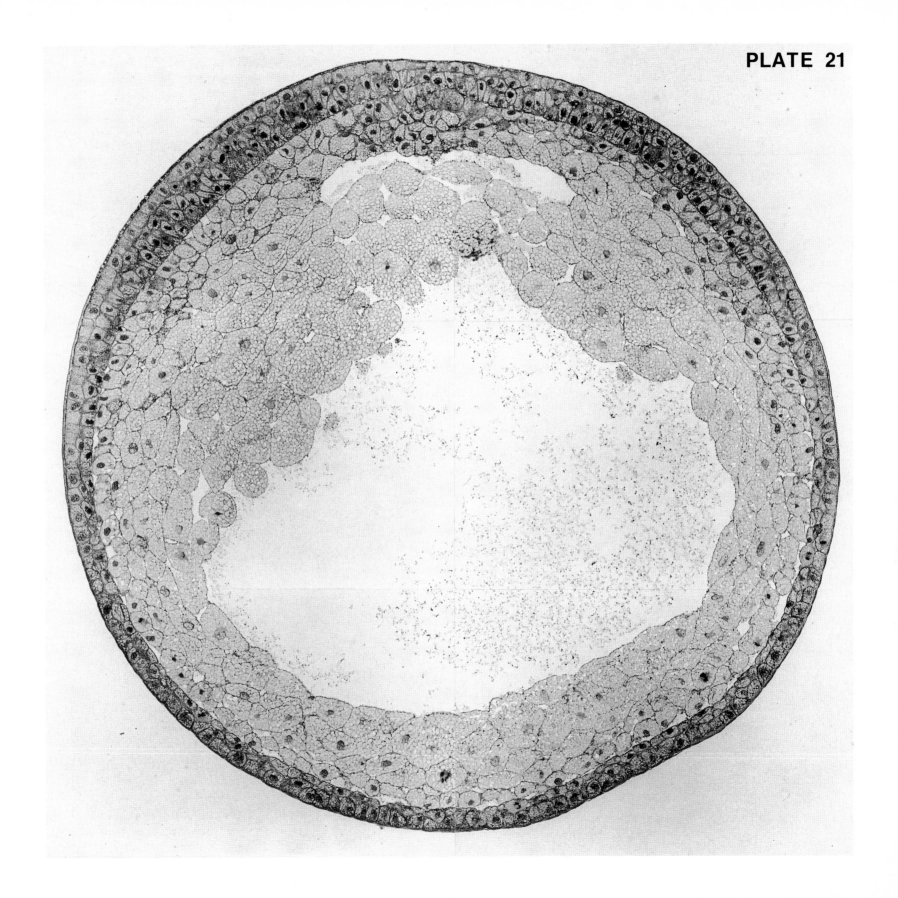

PLATE 21

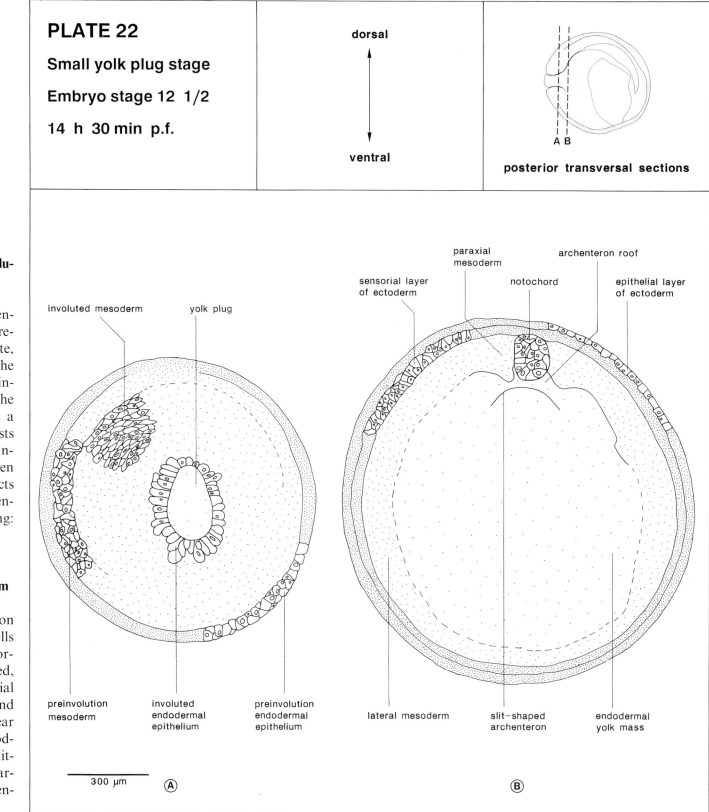

PLATE 22

Small yolk plug stage

Embryo stage 12 1/2

14 h 30 min p.f.

dorsal

ventral

posterior transversal sections

A B

A Cell Arrangement within the Zone of Involution

The section passes through the prospective endodermal epithelium twice. The outer layer represents this epithelium in its preinvolution state, the lining of the central yolk plug represents the prospective endodermal epithelium in its postinvolution state. In the subepithelial region the preinvolution prospective mesoderm exhibits a disordered cell arrangement, which contrasts with the whirl-like tangential order of the postinvolution mesodermal cells. This order, best seen on the *left side* of the section, probably reflects the movement of the involuted cells as they engage in circumferential intercalation. (Staining: BCB)

B The Structure of the Postinvolution Mesoderm

The section passes through the posterior region of the embryo slightly in front of the bottle cells at the tip of the ventral archenteron. In the dorsal mesoderm the notochord is clearly delimited, flanked on either side by converging paraxial mesoderm. The mesoderm extends laterally and thins out a little in the ventral region. No clear border separates the lateral and ventral mesoderm from the endodermal yolk mass. The slit-shaped archenteron is visible dorsally. The archenteron roof is formed by the involuted endodermal epithelium. (Staining: BCB)

involuted mesoderm

yolk plug

preinvolution mesoderm

involuted endodermal epithelium

preinvolution endodermal epithelium

300 μm

Ⓐ

sensorial layer of ectoderm

paraxial mesoderm

notochord

archenteron roof

epithelial layer of ectoderm

lateral mesoderm

slit-shaped archenteron

endodermal yolk mass

Ⓑ

PLATE 22

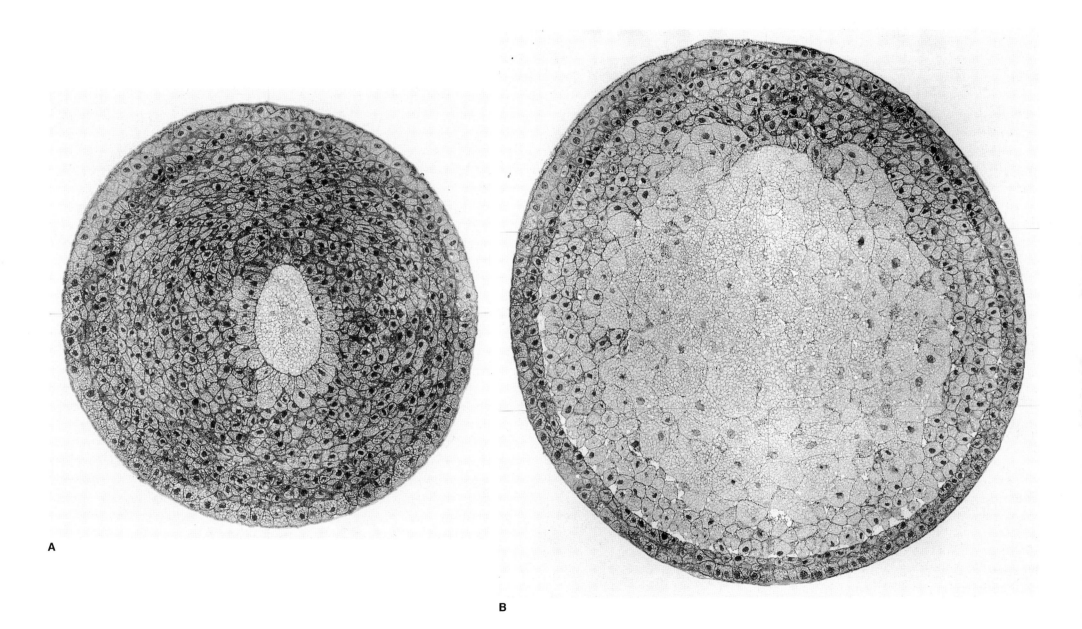

A

B

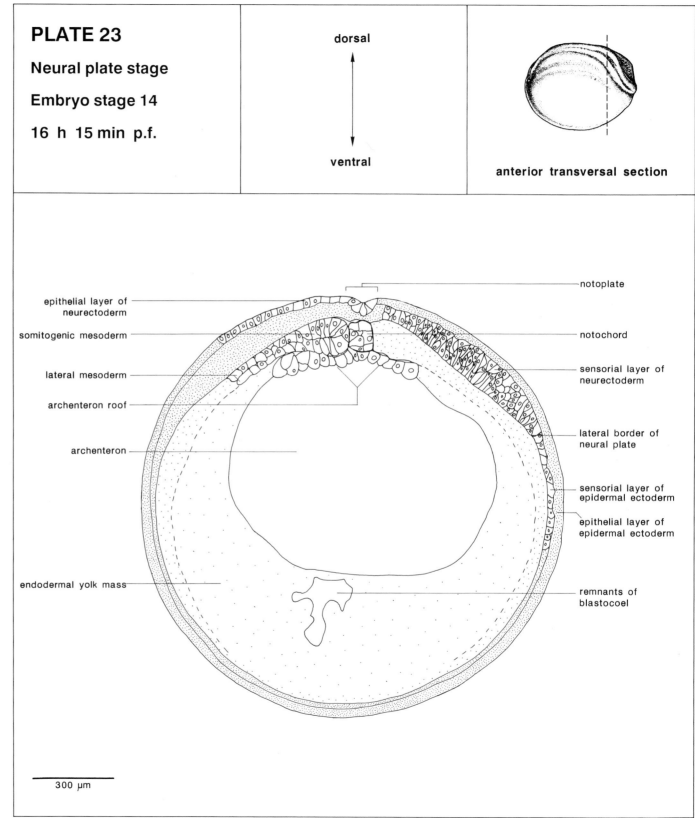

PLATE 23

Neural plate stage

Embryo stage 14

16 h 15 min p.f.

dorsal

ventral

anterior transversal section

notoplate

epithelial layer of
neurectoderm

somitogenic mesoderm

notochord

lateral mesoderm

sensorial layer of
neurectoderm

archenteron roof

archenteron

lateral border of
neural plate

sensorial layer of
epidermal ectoderm

epithelial layer of
epidermal ectoderm

endodermal yolk mass

remnants of
blastocoel

300 µm

The Neural Plate

The sensorial layer of the neurectoderm has become several cell layers thick in its lateral portions, in the center the region of the notoplate remains thinner. Bottle cell formation in this region indicates the onset of neural groove formation. Lateral to the neurectoderm the cells of the sensorial layer of the epidermal ectoderm have become very flat, compensating for the thickening of the neural plate by dorsal convergence.

The structures of the axial mesoderm are well segregated. The notochord is enveloped by the notochordal sheath. The paraxial material shows the typical double-layered arrangement of the somitogenic mesoderm. The lateral mesoderm begins to separate into two distinct layers and becomes segregated from the endodermal yolk mass. The blastocoel has largely disappeared. The cells of the archenteron roof differ in morphology from those lining the archenteron laterally and ventrally. (Staining: BCB)

PLATE 23

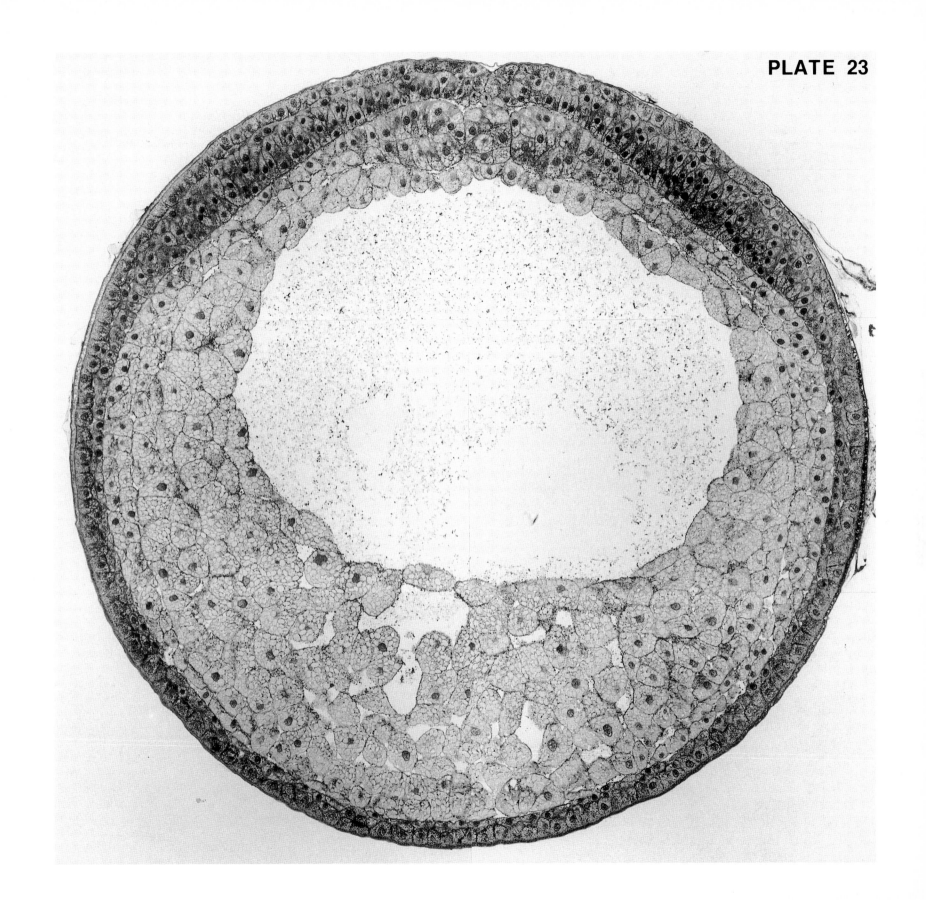

PLATE 24

Mid neural fold stage

Embryo early stage 15

17 h p.f.

dorsal

posterior ← → anterior

ventral

sagittal section

Neurula

The sensorial layer of the neural plate is markedly thickened in the anterior region. A clear border separates the anterior neurectoderm from the epidermal ectoderm.

The distribution of mesodermal material shows a marked dorsoventral asymmetry. The circumblastoporal collar harbors a massive accumulation of mesodermal cells. From this region dorsal axial mesoderm is continuously generated by radial intercalation and convergent extension. More to the anterior, the axial cells gradually assume a more regular arrangement as they form the notochord. The prechordal plate is represented by a thin layer of mesoderm underneath the anterior neural plate. Ventral to the anterior neural plate and the tip of the prechordal plate, a mesoderm-free zone allows direct contact between endodermal cells and the ectoderm. The stomodeum and the cement gland will form in this region. The archenteron is large dorsally and begins to bend ventrally in its anterior part. Ventrally, the archenteron has not significantly advanced, with bottle cells still present at its tip. A thin layer of spreading mesodermal cells separates the ventral ectoderm from the endodermal yolk mass. (Staining: BCB)

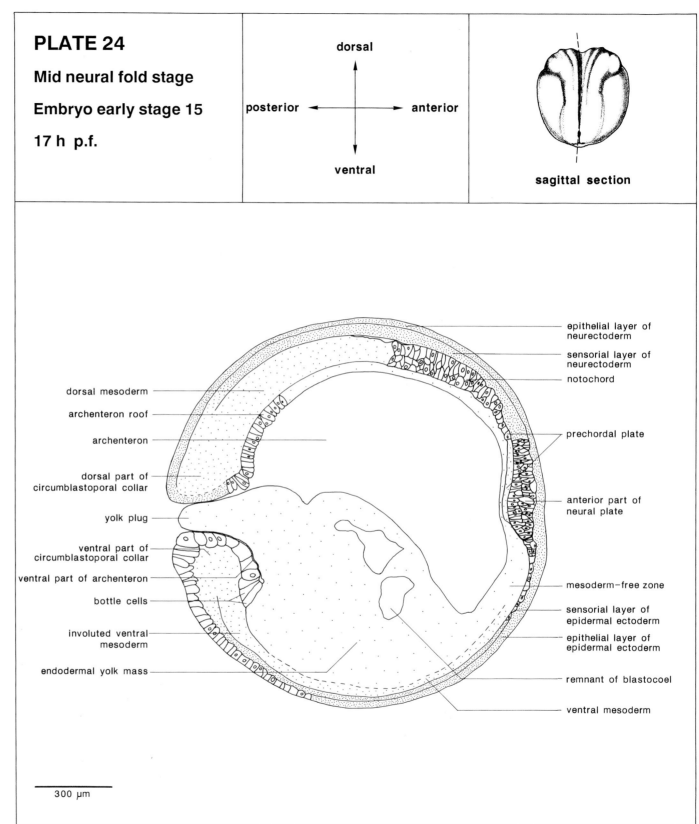

epithelial layer of neurectoderm

sensorial layer of neurectoderm

notochord

dorsal mesoderm

archenteron roof

archenteron

prechordal plate

dorsal part of circumblastoporal collar

yolk plug

anterior part of neural plate

ventral part of circumblastoporal collar

ventral part of archenteron

bottle cells

mesoderm-free zone

sensorial layer of epidermal ectoderm

epithelial layer of epidermal ectoderm

involuted ventral mesoderm

endodermal yolk mass

remnant of blastocoel

ventral mesoderm

300 µm

PLATE 24

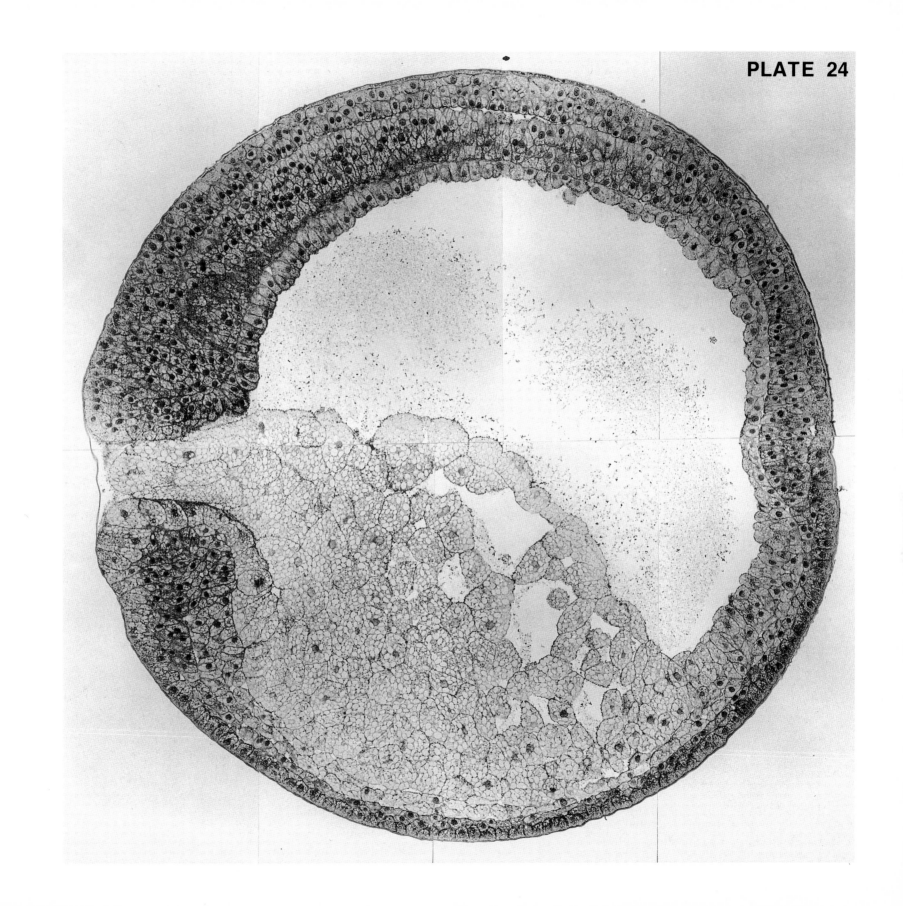

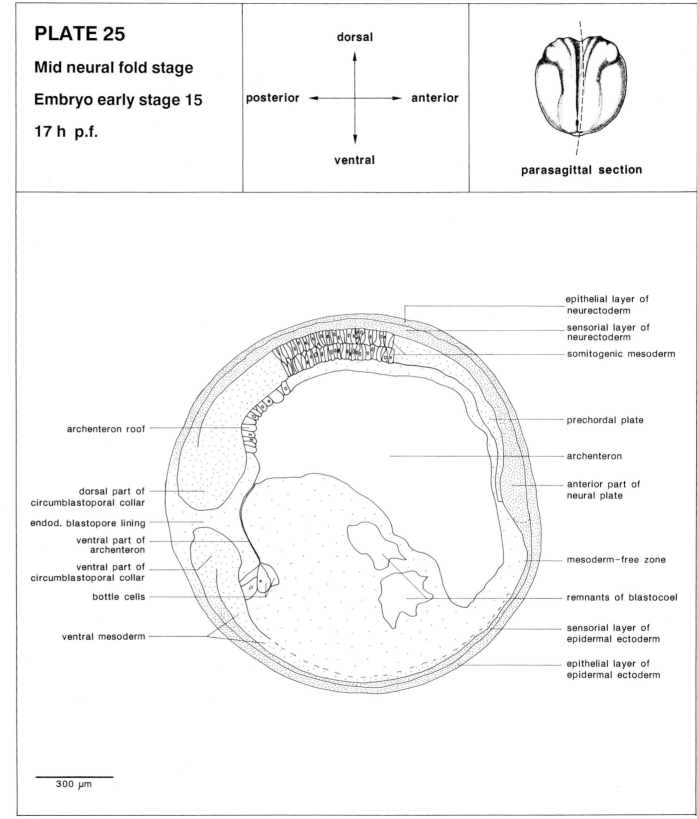

PLATE 25

Mid neural fold stage

Embryo early stage 15

17 h p.f.

dorsal

posterior ← → anterior

ventral

parasagittal section

epithelial layer of
neurectoderm

sensorial layer of
neurectoderm

somitogenic mesoderm

prechordal plate

archenteron

archenteron roof

anterior part of
neural plate

dorsal part of
circumblastoporal collar

endod. blastopore lining

ventral part of
archenteron

ventral part of
circumblastoporal collar

bottle cells

mesoderm−free zone

remnants of blastocoel

sensorial layer of
epidermal ectoderm

ventral mesoderm

epithelial layer of
epidermal ectoderm

300 µm

Neurula

This section is taken from the same specimen as
that on PLATE 24, but more laterally. Note the
double-layered cell arrangement within the somitogenic paraxial mesoderm. (Staining: BCB)

PLATE 25

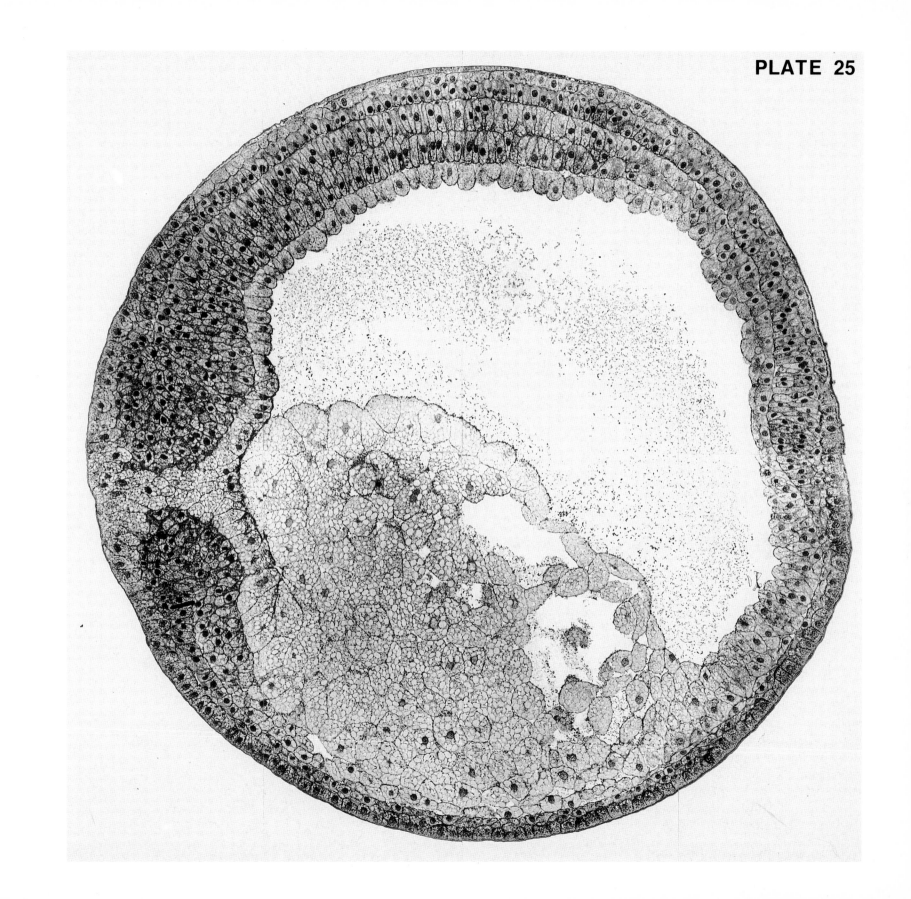

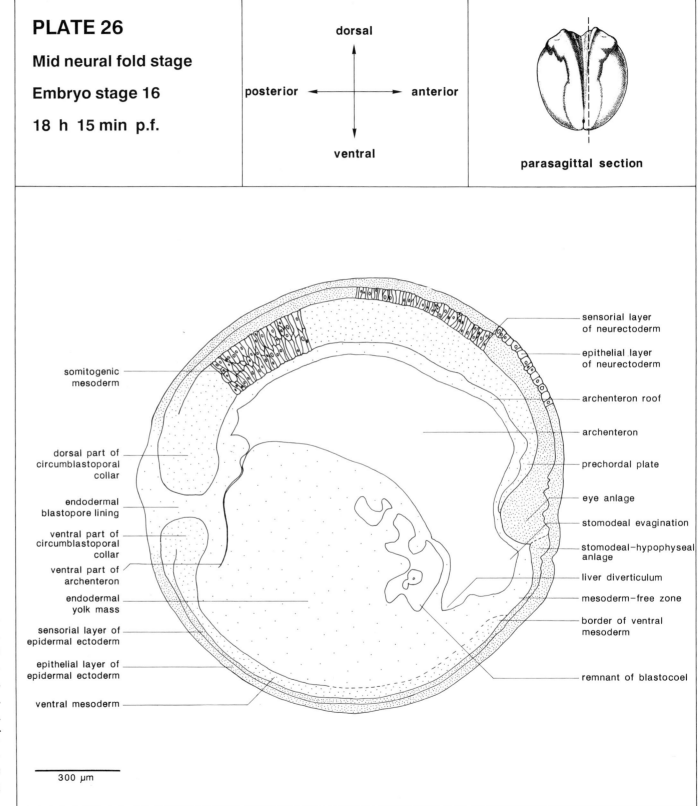

PLATE 26

Mid neural fold stage

Embryo stage 16

18 h 15 min p.f.

dorsal

posterior ← → anterior

ventral

parasagittal section

sensorial layer
of neurectoderm

epithelial layer
of neurectoderm

somitogenic
mesoderm

archenteron roof

archenteron

dorsal part of
circumblastoporal
collar

prechordal plate

eye anlage

endodermal
blastopore lining

stomodeal evagination

ventral part of
circumblastoporal
collar

stomodeal-hypophyseal
anlage

ventral part of
archenteron

liver diverticulum

endodermal
yolk mass

mesoderm-free zone

border of ventral
mesoderm

sensorial layer of
epidermal ectoderm

epithelial layer of
epidermal ectoderm

remnant of blastocoel

ventral mesoderm

300 µm

The Beginning of Eye Development

The eye anlage bulges from the anterior neural
plate. Ventral to the eye anlage the placodal
thickening of the stomodeal-hypophyseal anlage
has formed in the sensorial layer of the ectoderm. Within the somitogenic paraxial mesoderm vertical cell orientation is most conspicuous. Toward the circumblastoporal collar cell arrangement becomes chaotic. A thin layer of
spreading cells constitutes the ventral mesoderm.
The anterior archenteron bends ventrally. The
stomodeal evagination and the liver diverticulum
begin to form. (Staining: BCB)

PLATE 26

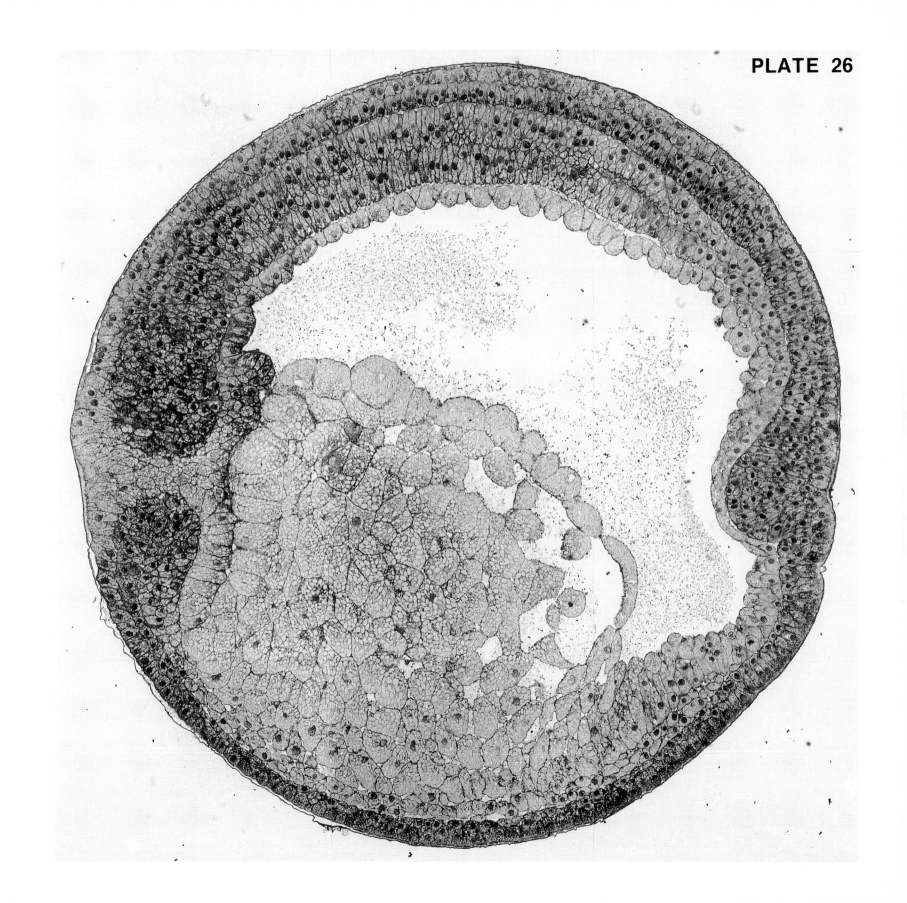

PLATE 27

Mid neural fold stage

Embryo stage 16

18 h 15 min p.f.

dorsal

↕

ventral

anterior transversal section

Neural Tube Formation in the Head Region at the Level of the Rhombencephalon

Bottle cells have formed in the epithelial layer of the notoplate region. As they invaginate to form the neural groove, lateral epithelial cells are drawn toward the midline. The cell arrangement in the sensorial layer allows the subdivision of the neural plate into a central region and the lateral regions. In the central region the neurogenic cells orient mediolaterally to participate in neural tube formation. Laterally the disordered arrangement of the cells indicates their belonging to the neural crest.

The dorsal rim of the paraxial somitogenic mesoderm is lifted above the level of the notochord, a change in shape which supports neural tube closure. The lateral plate mesoderm consists of two layers: the outer, prospective somatic (or parietal) and the inner, prospective splanchnic (or visceral) layer. Note the difference in cell morphology between the dorsal archenteron roof and the lateral and ventral lining of the archenteron. (Staining: BCB)

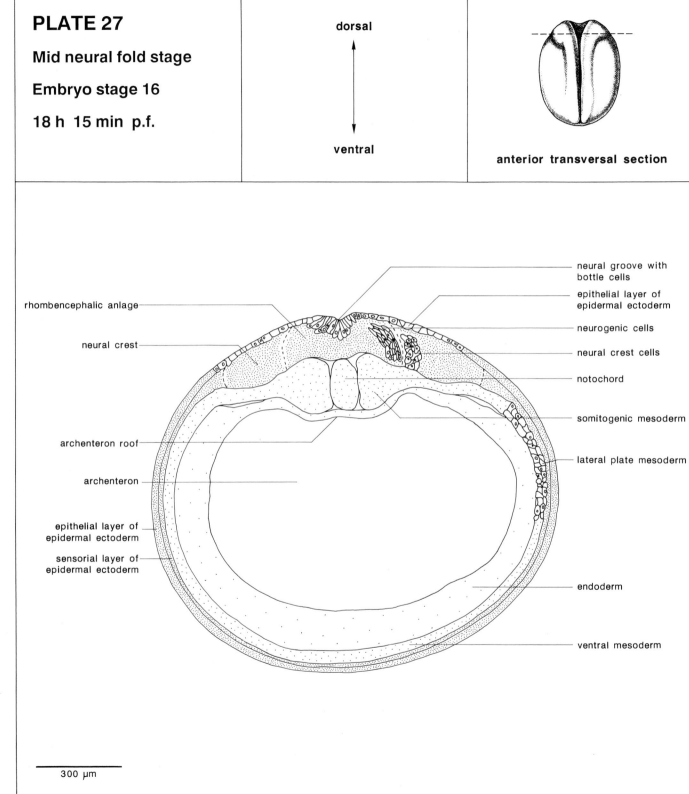

rhombencephalic anlage

neural crest

archenteron roof

archenteron

epithelial layer of epidermal ectoderm

sensorial layer of epidermal ectoderm

neural groove with bottle cells

epithelial layer of epidermal ectoderm

neurogenic cells

neural crest cells

notochord

somitogenic mesoderm

lateral plate mesoderm

endoderm

ventral mesoderm

300 µm

PLATE 27

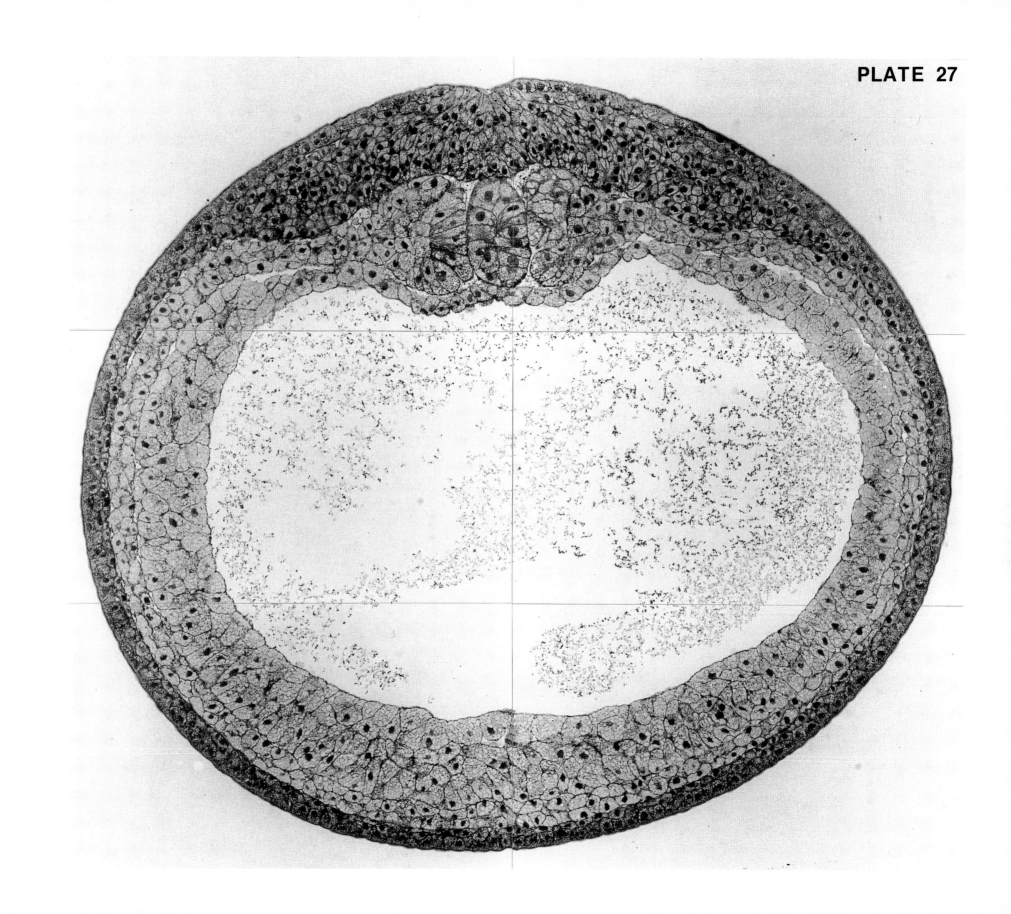

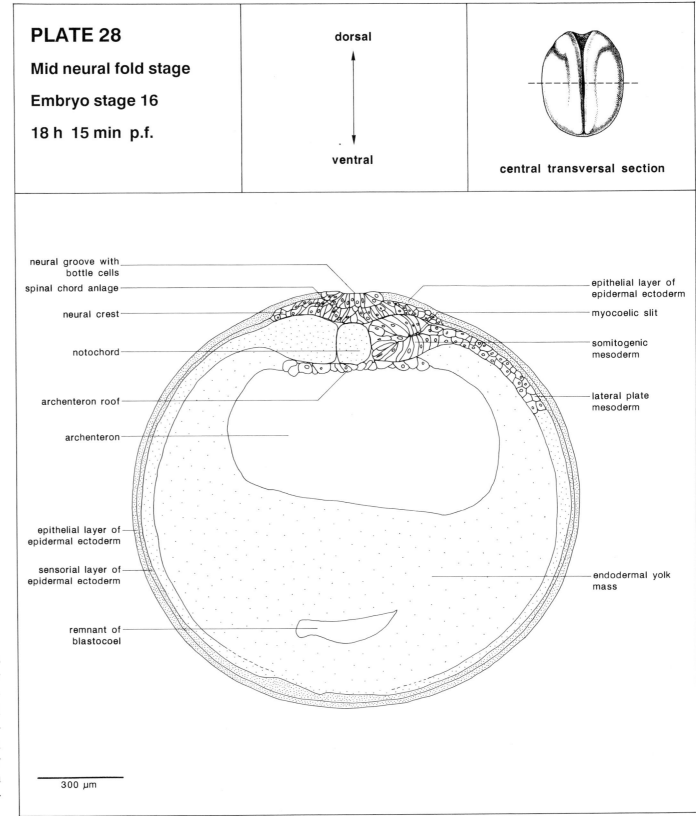

PLATE 28

Mid neural fold stage

Embryo stage 16

18 h 15 min p.f.

dorsal

ventral

central transversal section

neural groove with bottle cells

spinal chord anlage

neural crest

notochord

archenteron roof

archenteron

epithelial layer of epidermal ectoderm

sensorial layer of epidermal ectoderm

remnant of blastocoel

epithelial layer of epidermal ectoderm

myocoelic slit

somitogenic mesoderm

lateral plate mesoderm

endodermal yolk mass

300 µm

Neural Tube Formation in the Trunk Region

The pattern of orientation of the neurogenic cells of the prospective spinal chord indicates their convergence toward the midline. Bottle cell formation in the epithelial layer of the neural groove is prominent. Compared to the head region the number of neural crest cells present in the lateral part of the neural plate is significantly smaller. The other features are similar to those in PLATE 27. Note the myocoelic slit in the somitogenic mesoderm. (Staining: BCB)

PLATE 28

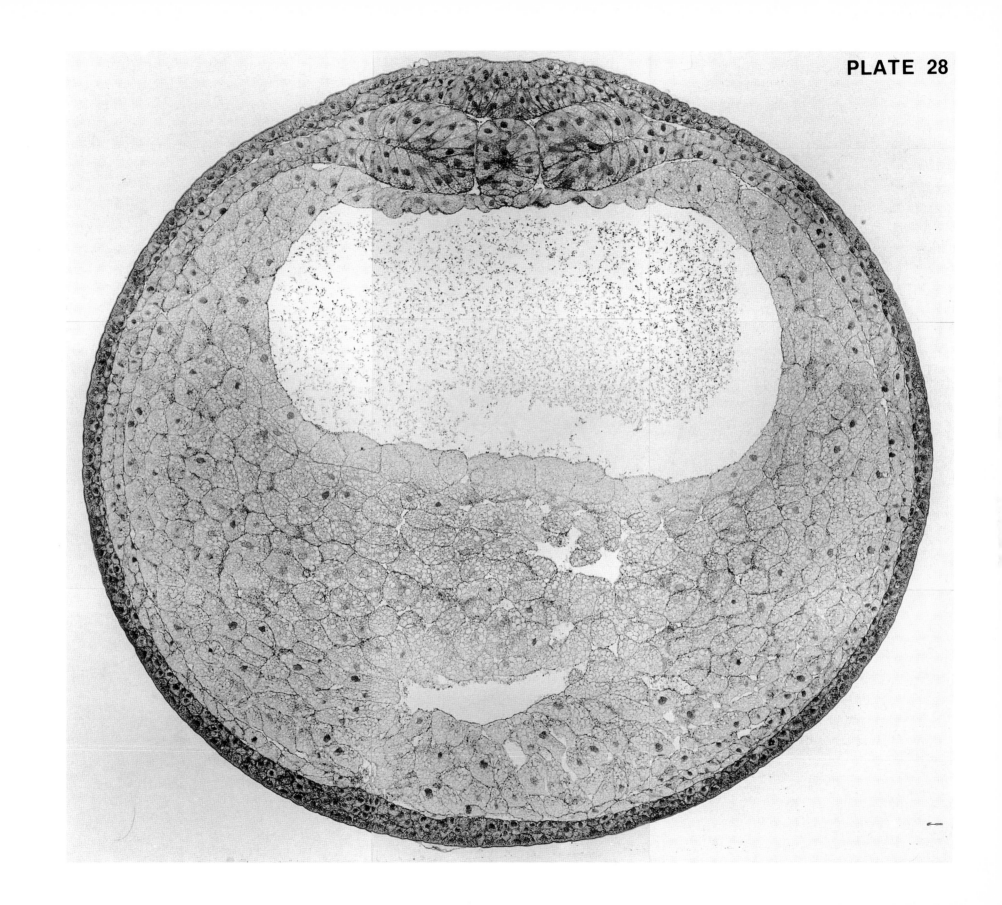

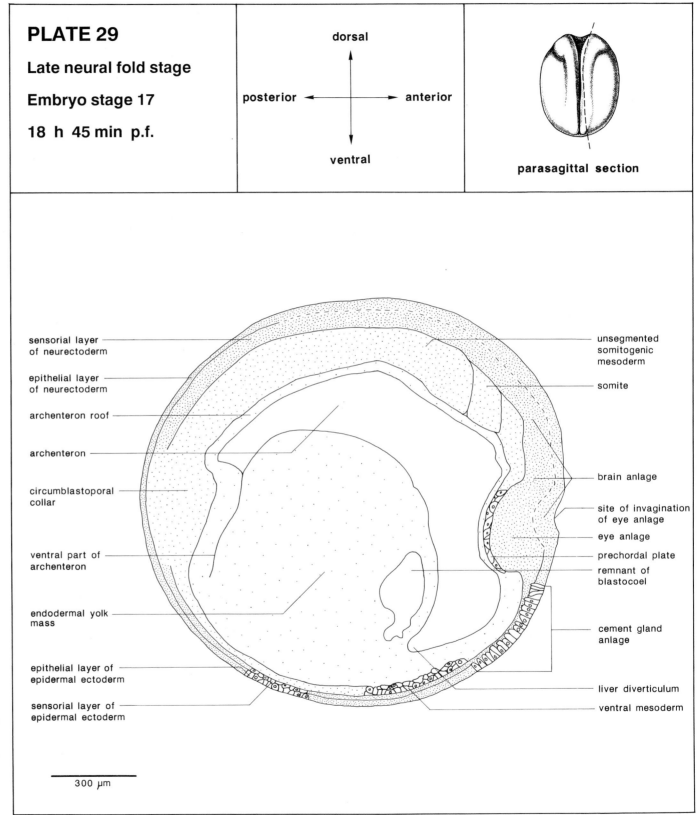

PLATE 29

Late neural fold stage

Embryo stage 17

18 h 45 min p.f.

dorsal

posterior ← → anterior

ventral

parasagittal section

sensorial layer
of neurectoderm

epithelial layer
of neurectoderm

archenteron roof

archenteron

circumblastoporal
collar

ventral part of
archenteron

endodermal yolk
mass

epithelial layer of
epidermal ectoderm

sensorial layer of
epidermal ectoderm

unsegmented
somitogenic
mesoderm

somite

brain anlage

site of invagination
of eye anlage

eye anlage

prechordal plate

remnant of
blastocoel

cement gland
anlage

liver diverticulum

ventral mesoderm

300 µm

The Onset of Somitogenesis

The first three somites have segregated from the paraxial mesoderm. Further material is constantly added to the axial mesoderm from the circumblastoporal region. The ventral mesoderm is represented by a thin double-layered sheet of cells.

The eye anlage has formed in the prosencephalic region of the brain and begins to invaginate. Dorsal convergence of the sensorial layer of the neurectoderm has led to the marked thickening of the neural anlage. Between the anterior end of the brain anlage and the border of the ventral mesoderm the cells of the epithelial layer of the ectoderm columnarize to form the anlage of the cement gland. The liver diverticulum has deepened and extends ventrally. (Staining: BCB)

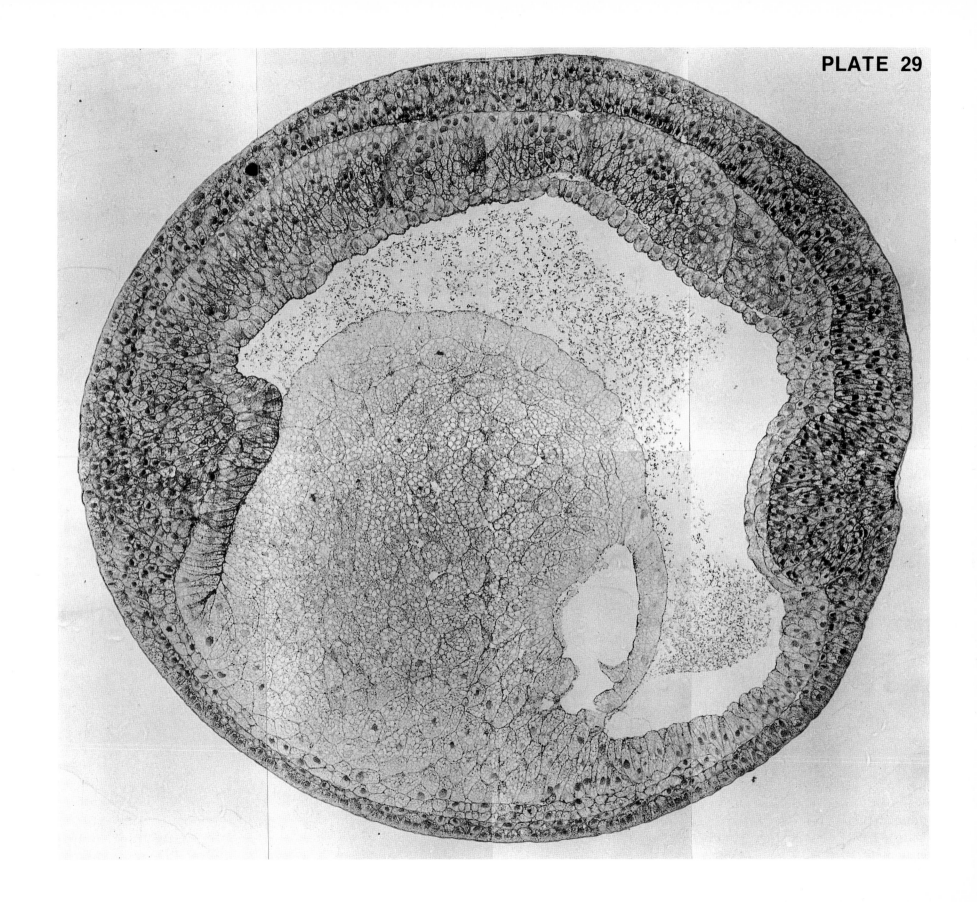

PLATE 29

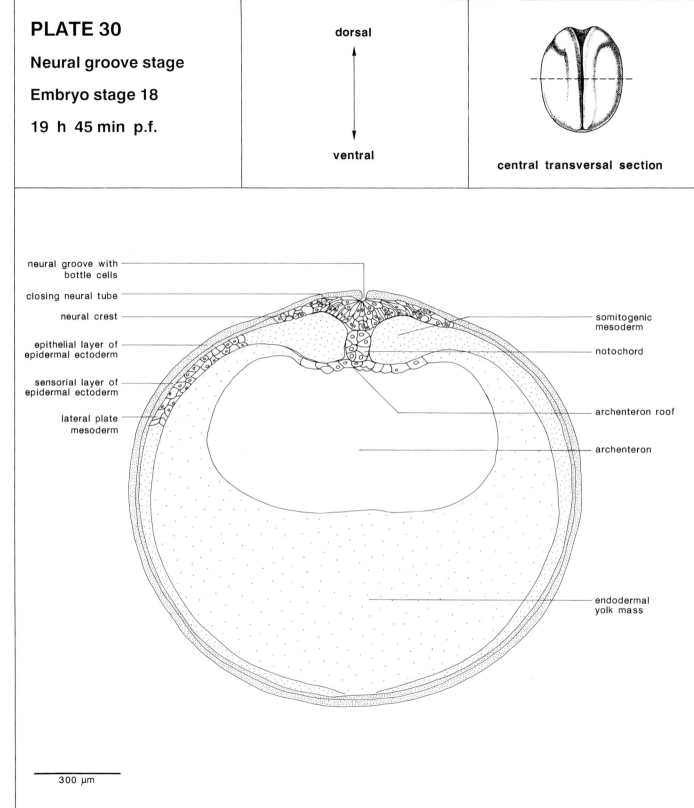

PLATE 30

Neural groove stage

Embryo stage 18

19 h 45 min p.f.

dorsal

ventral

central transversal section

neural groove with bottle cells

closing neural tube

neural crest

epithelial layer of epidermal ectoderm

sensorial layer of epidermal ectoderm

lateral plate mesoderm

somitogenic mesoderm

notochord

archenteron roof

archenteron

endodermal yolk mass

300 μm

Neural Tube Closure

The bottle cells of the neural groove have moved to the inside and the lateral epithelial layer moves over the neural tube which is about to close. Within the neural tube the cells have oriented toward the center. The notochord keeps close contact with the neural tube floor. The massive somitogenic mesoderm supports neural tube closure by lifting the lateral neurectoderm. The lateral plate mesoderm is double-layered. The smooth lining of the archenteron might indicate the presence of an epithelium. The cells at the center of the archenteron roof exhibit a different morphology. (Staining: BCB)

PLATE 30

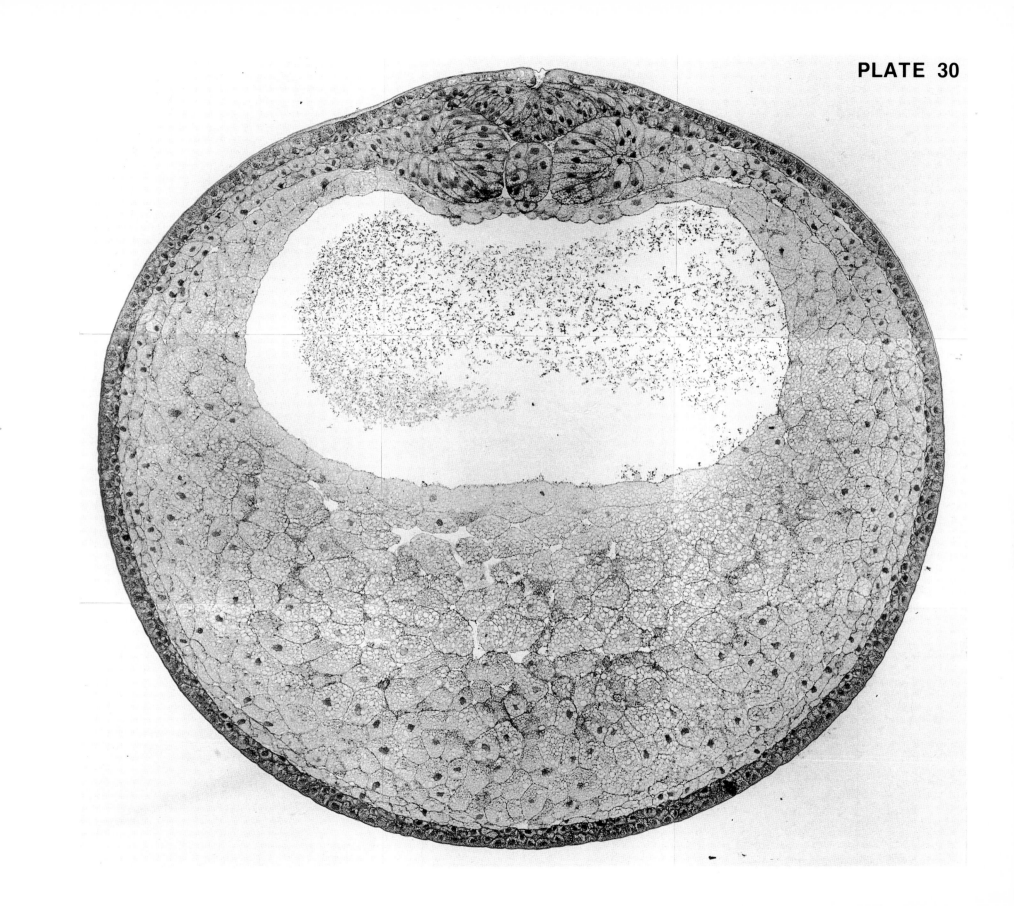

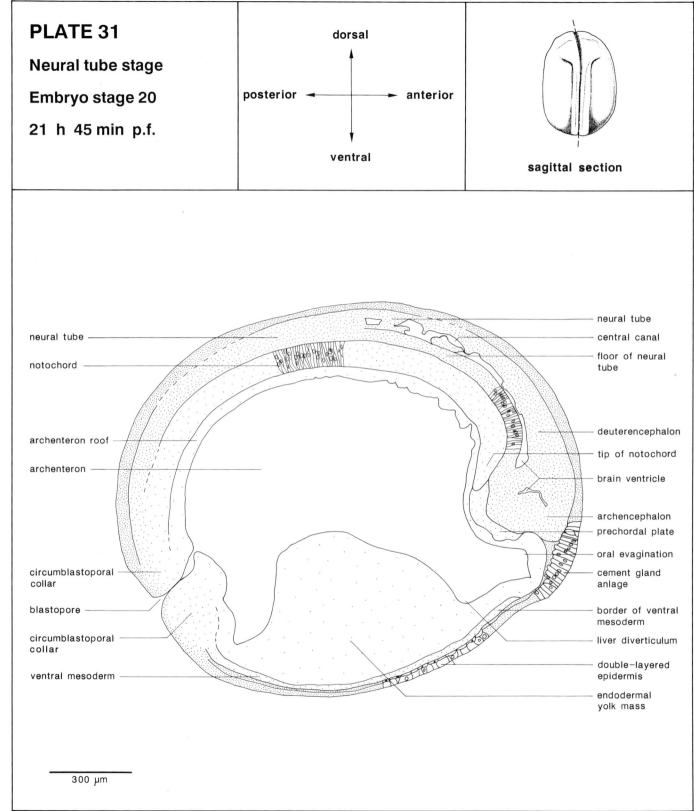

PLATE 31

Neural tube stage

Embryo stage 20

21 h 45 min p.f.

dorsal

posterior ← → anterior

ventral

sagittal section

Cell Arrangement in the Notochord

The differentiation of the axial mesoderm proceeds asynchronously along the anterior-posterior axis, such that the anterior region exhibits the more advanced stages and the posterior region the "younger" stages, which have just emerged from the blastoporal collar. This section shows the structural changes of the notochord with advancing age. In the circumblastoporal region mesodermal and neurogenic cells cannot be distinguished. As one moves anteriorly the boundary between the notochord and the ectodermal and endodermal tissues sharpens, and the cells within the notochord flatten and assume a stacked arrangement. In the head region the notochord tapers and ends in the prechordal plate mesoderm.

The brain becomes subdivided into the archencephalic and the deuterencephalic region. The neural tube encloses the central canal. The anlage of the cement gland protrudes as the cells of the epithelial layer of the ectoderm become columnar. The oral evagination is a prominent feature of the anterior archenteron. In this embryo the archenteron is exceptionally inflated. Other features of the embryo are not affected by this aberrant property. (Staining: BCB)

neural tube

notochord

archenteron roof

archenteron

circumblastoporal collar

blastopore

circumblastoporal collar

ventral mesoderm

neural tube

central canal

floor of neural tube

deuterencephalon

tip of notochord

brain ventricle

archencephalon

prechordal plate

oral evagination

cement gland anlage

border of ventral mesoderm

liver diverticulum

double-layered epidermis

endodermal yolk mass

300 μm

PLATE 31

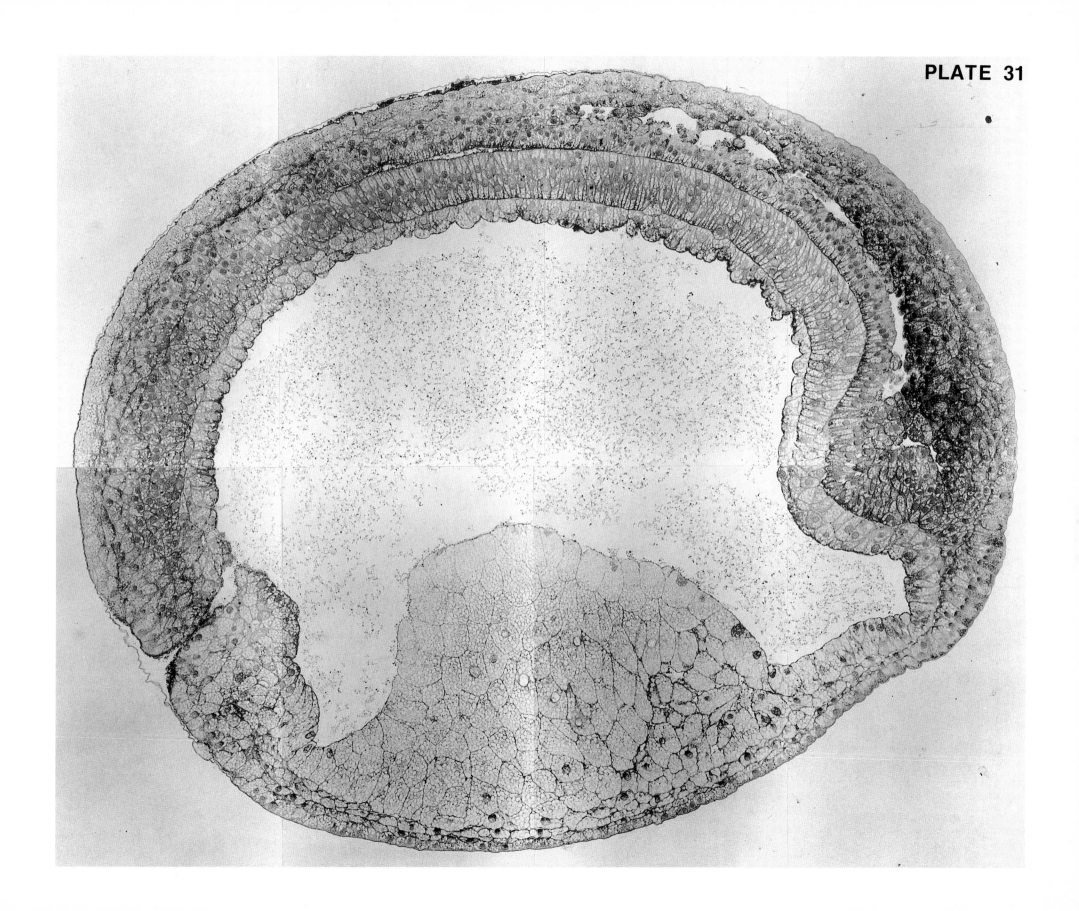

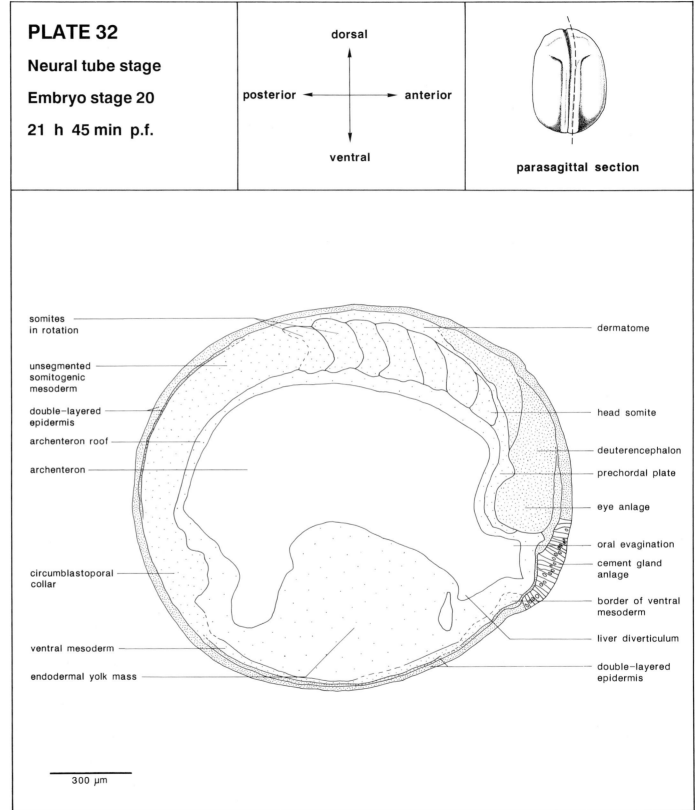

PLATE 32

Neural tube stage

Embryo stage 20

21 h 45 min p.f.

dorsal

posterior ← → anterior

ventral

parasagittal section

somites in rotation

unsegmented somitogenic mesoderm

double-layered epidermis

archenteron roof

archenteron

circumblastoporal collar

ventral mesoderm

endodermal yolk mass

dermatome

head somite

deuterencephalon

prechordal plate

eye anlage

oral evagination

cement gland anlage

border of ventral mesoderm

liver diverticulum

double-layered epidermis

300 µm

Somite Formation Continued

Six somites have segregated from the paraxial mesoderm, the seventh is in the process of rotation. The subdivision of the brain anlage is most conspicuous in this section. For further explanation see text to PLATE 31, which shows the adjacent sagittal section. (Staining: BCB)

PLATE 32

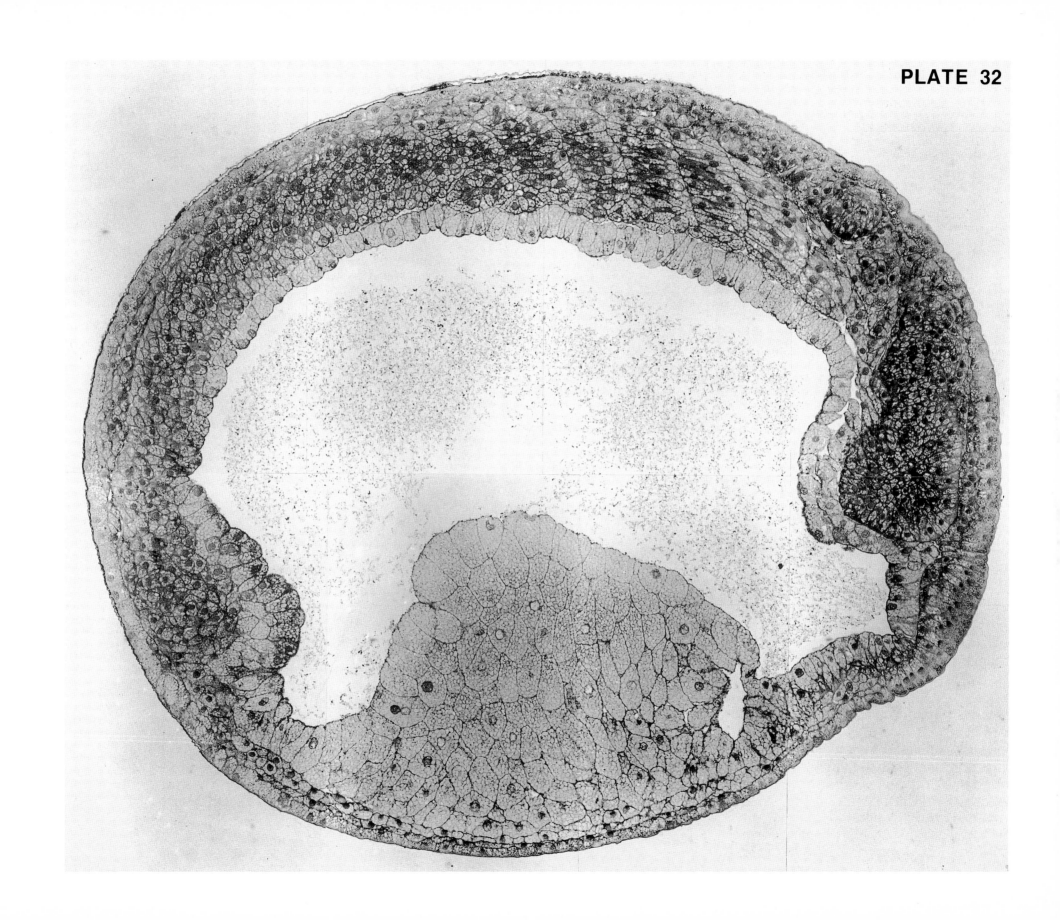

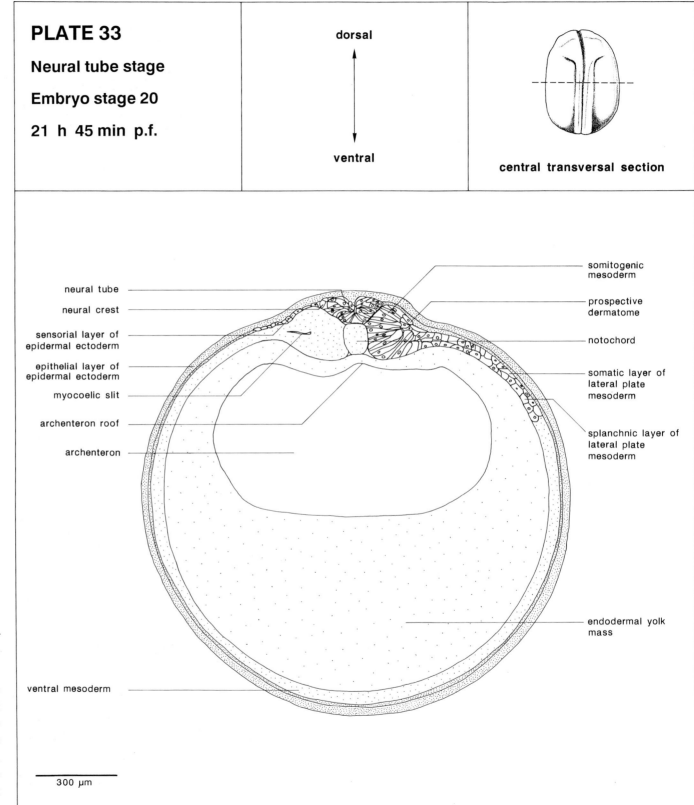

PLATE 33

Neural tube stage

Embryo stage 20

21 h 45 min p.f.

dorsal

ventral

central transversal section

somitogenic
mesoderm

neural tube

prospective
dermatome

neural crest

sensorial layer of
epidermal ectoderm

notochord

epithelial layer of
epidermal ectoderm

somatic layer of
lateral plate
mesoderm

myocoelic slit

archenteron roof

splanchnic layer of
lateral plate
mesoderm

archenteron

endodermal yolk
mass

ventral mesoderm

300 µm

Neural Tube Closed

The epithelial layer of epidermal ectoderm covers the neural tube completely. The two ridges of the somitogenic mesoderm have risen further above the level of the notochord, as the somitogenic cells are shifted toward the midline where they pile up horizontally at the notochord/neural tube border. This movement also contributes to the elevation of the axial structures above the originally circular outline of the embryo. Within the lateral plate mesoderm, the somatic and the splanchnic layers can be distinguished. (Staining: BCB)

PLATE 33

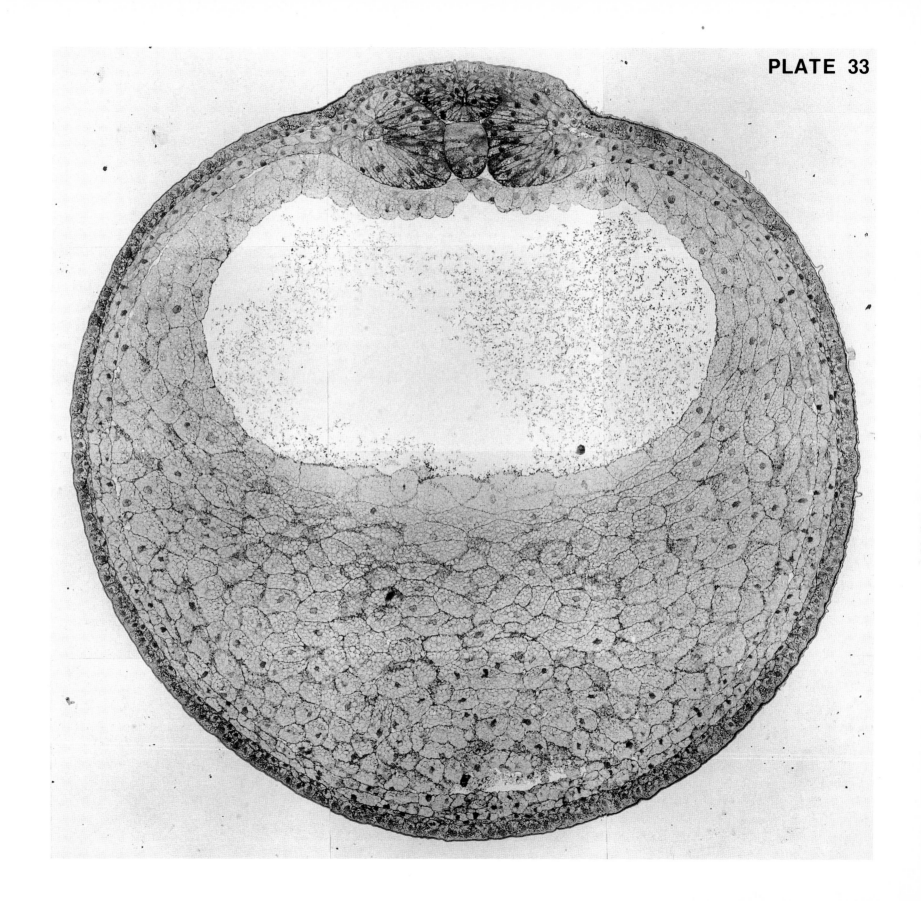

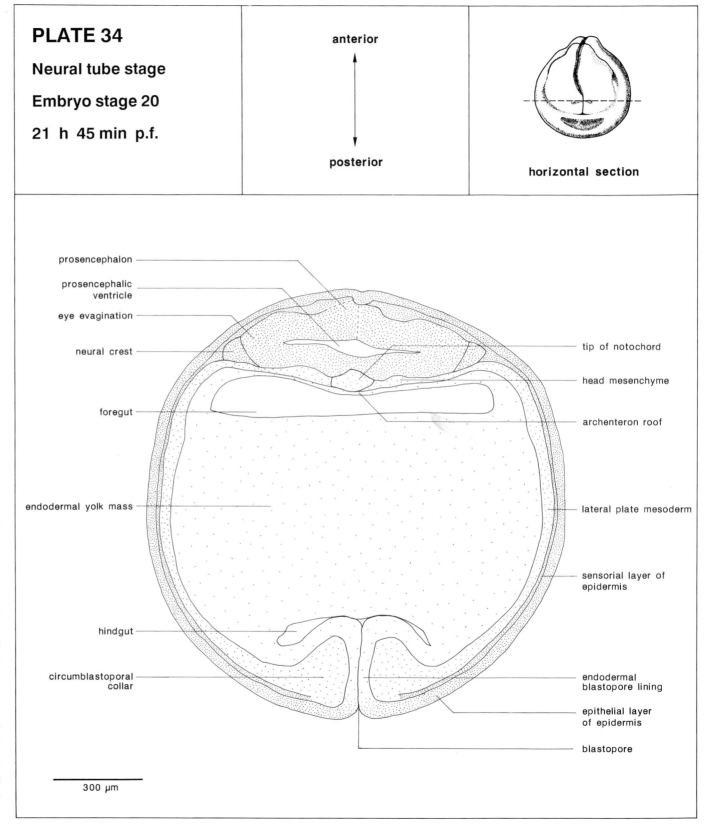

PLATE 34

Neural tube stage

Embryo stage 20

21 h 45 min p.f.

anterior

posterior

horizontal section

prosencephalon

prosencephalic
ventricle

eye evagination

neural crest

foregut

endodermal yolk mass

hindgut

circumblastoporal
collar

tip of notochord

head mesenchyme

archenteron roof

lateral plate mesoderm

sensorial layer of
epidermis

endodermal
blastopore lining

epithelial layer
of epidermis

blastopore

300 µm

Evagination of the Eye Vesicle from the Prosencephalic Region

This horizontal section passes through the blastopore region and the prosencephalon. The prosencephalon is characterized by the two lateral evaginations of the eye anlagen. The ventricular cavity extends through the prospective optic stalk into the eye vesicles. Lateral to the eye anlagen some of the anteriormost neural crest material is seen. The mesodermal cell aggregation beneath the center of the prosencephalon represents the anterior tip of the notochord. Note how the cells lining the foregut change shape as they adapt to the spatial requirements in this region. The epithelium lining the hindgut is continuous with the blastoporal lining and the epithelial layer of the posterior epidermis. (Staining: BCB)

PLATE 34

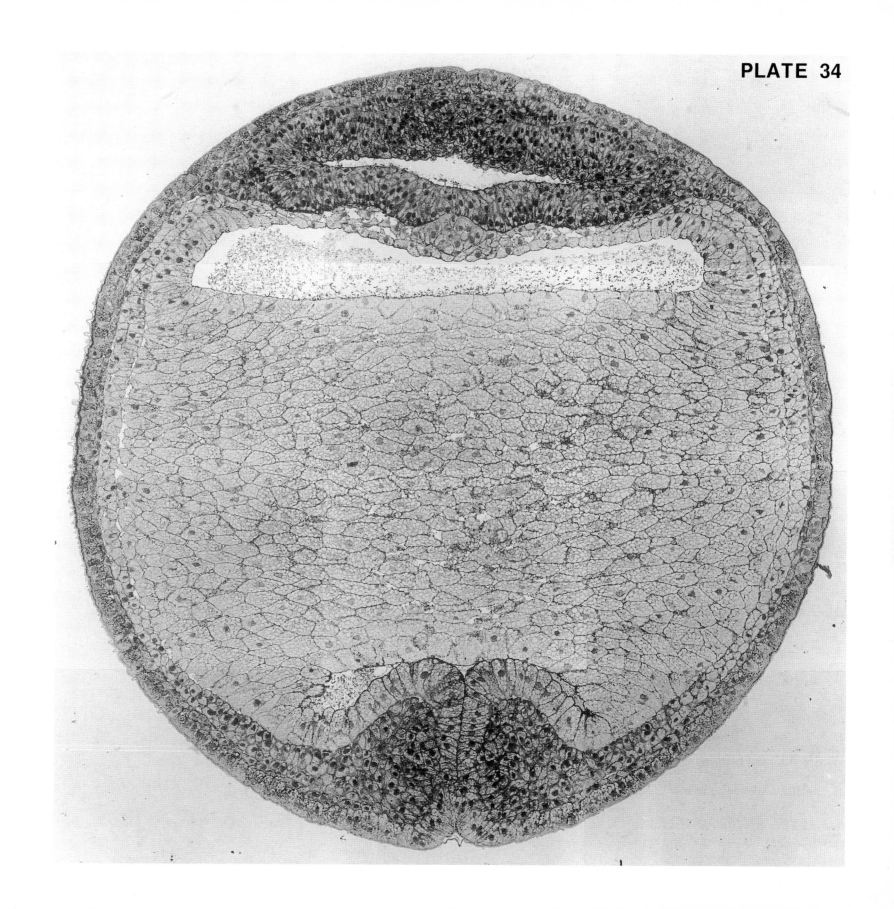

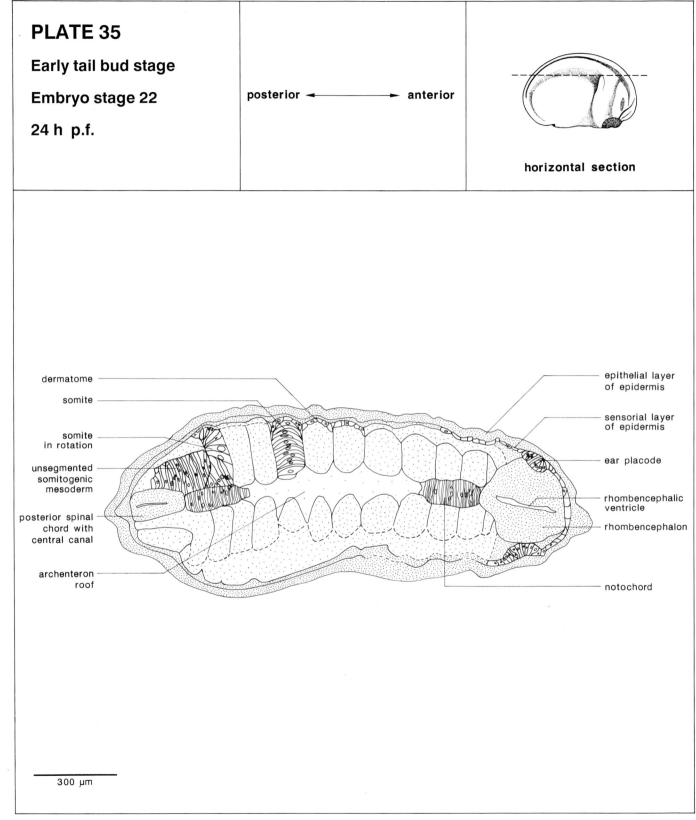

PLATE 35

Early tail bud stage

Embryo stage 22

24 h p.f.

posterior ←——————→ anterior

horizontal section

dermatome

somite

somite in rotation

unsegmented somitogenic mesoderm

posterior spinal chord with central canal

archenteron roof

epithelial layer of epidermis

sensorial layer of epidermis

ear placode

rhombencephalic ventricle

rhombencephalon

notochord

300 μm

The Somite Pattern

The midline of the section passes (from *right to left*) through the rhombencephalic region of the brain, the anterior notochord, some of the archenteron roof, the posterior notochord, and the spinal chord. Most of the paraxial mesoderm visible in this section is segmented into somites, the exact anterior-posterior alignment of their cells is most conspicuous. The dermatome, lateral to the somites, remains unsegmented and forms a continuous subepidermal layer in *Xenopus*. The ear placode has formed adjacent to the rhombencephalon in the sensorial layer of the head epidermis. (Staining: BCB)

PLATE 35

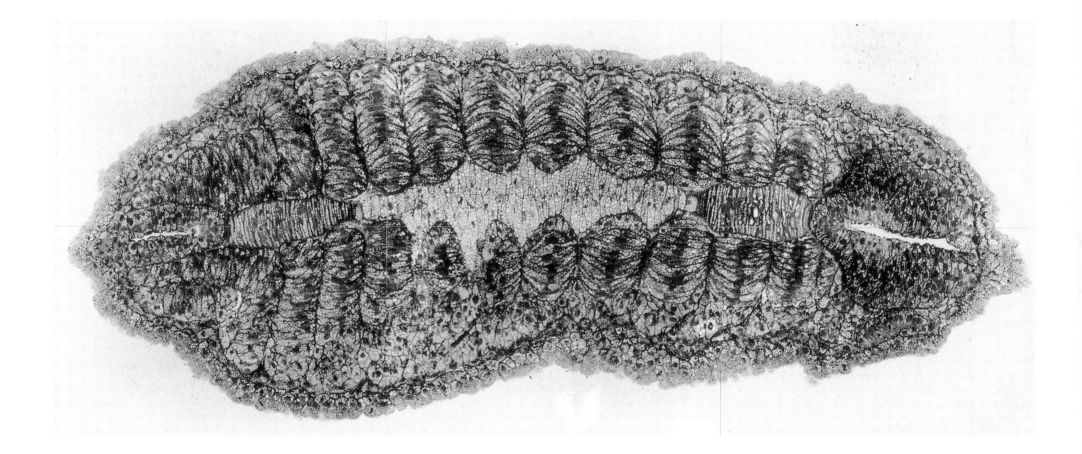

PLATE 36

Early tail bud stage

Embryo stage 23

1 d 45 min p.f.

dorsal

posterior ← → anterior

ventral

sagittal section

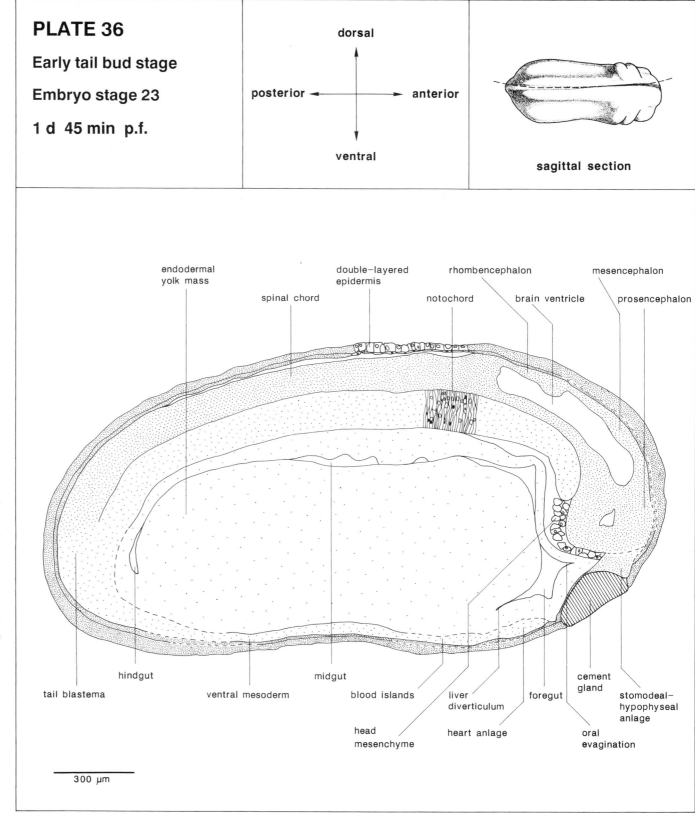

endodermal
yolk mass

spinal chord

double–layered
epidermis

rhombencephalon

mesencephalon

notochord

brain ventricle

prosencephalon

hindgut

midgut

cement
gland

tail blastema

ventral mesoderm

blood islands

liver
diverticulum

foregut

stomodeal–
hypophyseal
anlage

head
mesenchyme

heart anlage

oral
evagination

300 µm

The Basic Body Pattern (I)

The vacuolization of the notochordal cells contributes to the stiffness of the notochord and to its longitudinal extension which causes a stretching of the body. As a result the endodermal yolk mass is pressed against the midgut which is reduced to a narrow slit. The liver diverticulum protrudes from the foregut in posterior direction. The oral evagination of the foregut narrows and approaches the stomodeal-hypophyseal anlage of the ectoderm. Due to the cephalic flexure the brain is bent. It is subdivided into pros-, mes-, and rhombencephalon; the brain ventricle is enlarged. The cells of the cement gland begin to accumulate their secretion product. In the posterior region of the embryo neural tube, notochord, and paraxial mesoderm emerge from the seemingly undifferentiated tail blastema. Blood islands and the heart anlage begin to form in the anterior-ventral mesoderm. (Staining: BCB)

PLATE 36

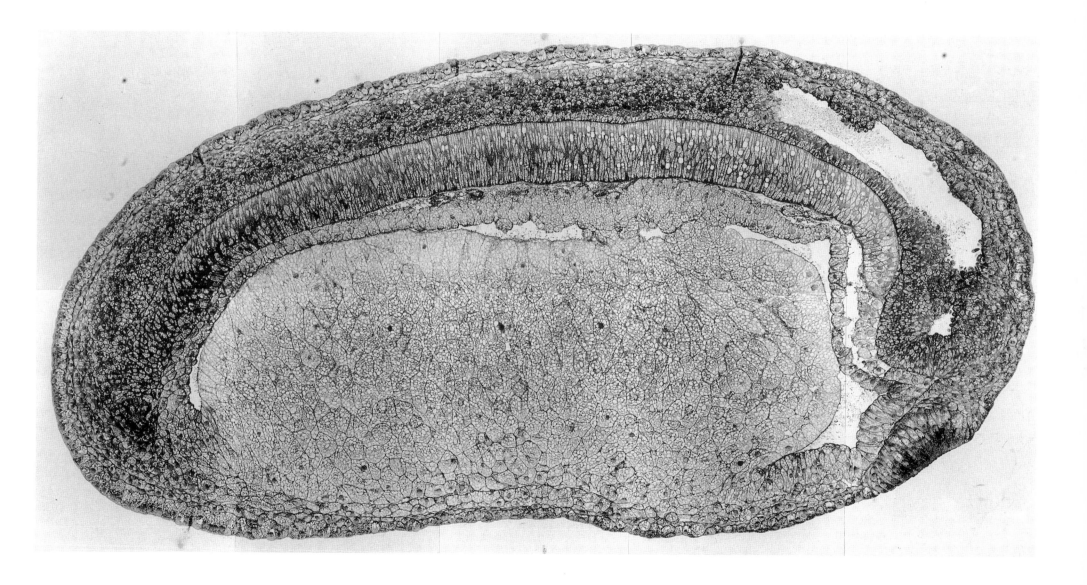

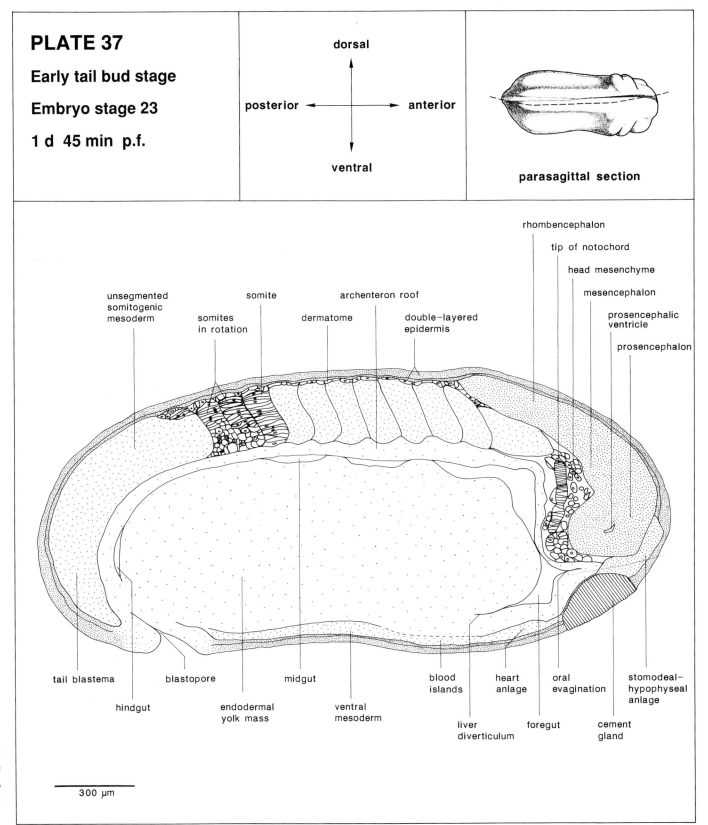

PLATE 37

Early tail bud stage

Embryo stage 23

1 d 45 min p.f.

dorsal

posterior ←——→ anterior

ventral

parasagittal section

rhombencephalon

tip of notochord

head mesenchyme

mesencephalon

prosencephalic ventricle

prosencephalon

unsegmented somitogenic mesoderm

somites in rotation

somite

dermatome

archenteron roof

double–layered epidermis

tail blastema

hindgut

blastopore

endodermal yolk mass

midgut

ventral mesoderm

blood islands

liver diverticulum

heart anlage

foregut

oral evagination

cement gland

stomodeal–hypophyseal anlage

300 µm

The Basic Body Pattern (II)

The paraxial mesoderm is in the process of segmentation; ten somites have formed. The hindgut extends posteriorly beyond the level of the blastopore. For further explanation see legend to PLATE 36, which shows the adjacent sagittal section. (Staining: BCB)

PLATE 37

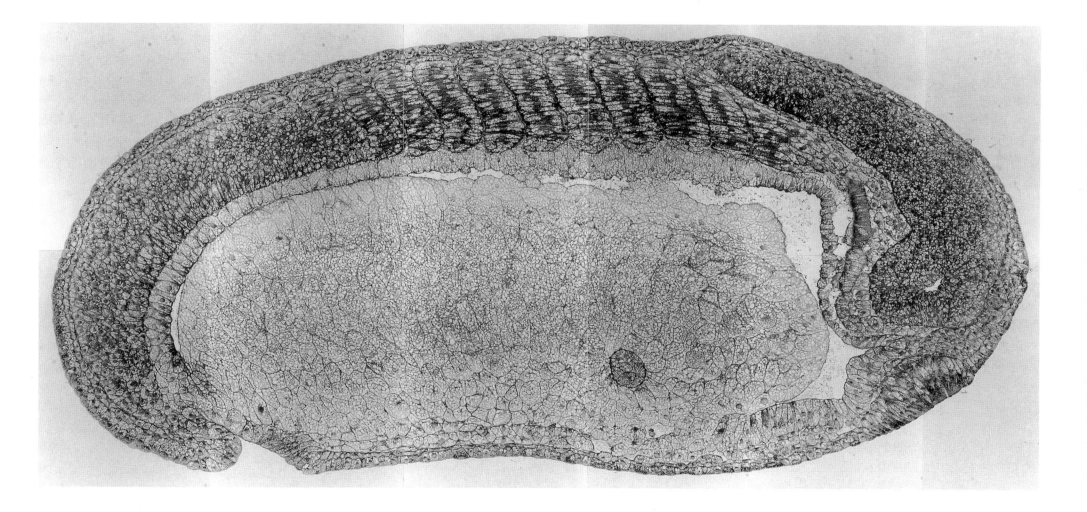

PLATE 38

Early tail bud stage

Embryo stage 23

1 d 45 min p.f.

dorsal

↕

ventral

transversal sections

A Formation of the Pronephric Anlage

In the anterior trunk region, cells of the somatic layer of the lateral plate have formed an aggregate which represents the pronephric anlage. The process of somite formation by rotation has been completed in the anterior half of the trunk (cf. PLATE 37). The section passes perpendicularly through the longitudinal axis of the spindle-shaped cells. The dermatome did not participate in the rotation and forms a thin layer separating the dorsolateral part of the somites from the epidermis. The cells of the outer epidermal layer show signs of differentiation. Mucus secreting glandular cells are present. (Staining: BCB)

B Eye Formation

Due to the bending of the brain (cf. PLATE 36), the section passes through the prosencephalon and the mesencephalon. The massive eye vesicles have evaginated from the prosencephalon and remain connected to the brain through the optic stalk. The brain ventricle extends into the eye vesicles. The walls of the eye vesicle can be divided into a thick ventrolateral portion, representing the prospective retinal layer, and a thinner dorsomedian portion, representing the prospective pigment layer of the retina (cf. PLATE 41). Neural crest material has migrated into the space between brain and eye vesicle. Laterally the eye vesicle is in close contact with the epidermis. The cement gland is a differentiation of the epithelial layer of the epidermis. The very thin sensorial layer separates the gland from the underlying head mesenchyme. (Staining: BCB)

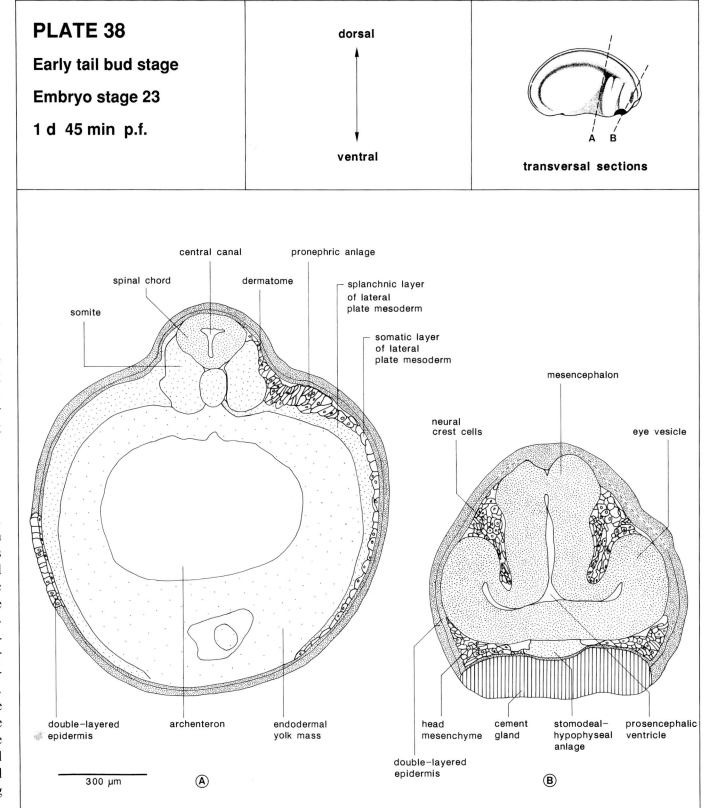

PLATE 38

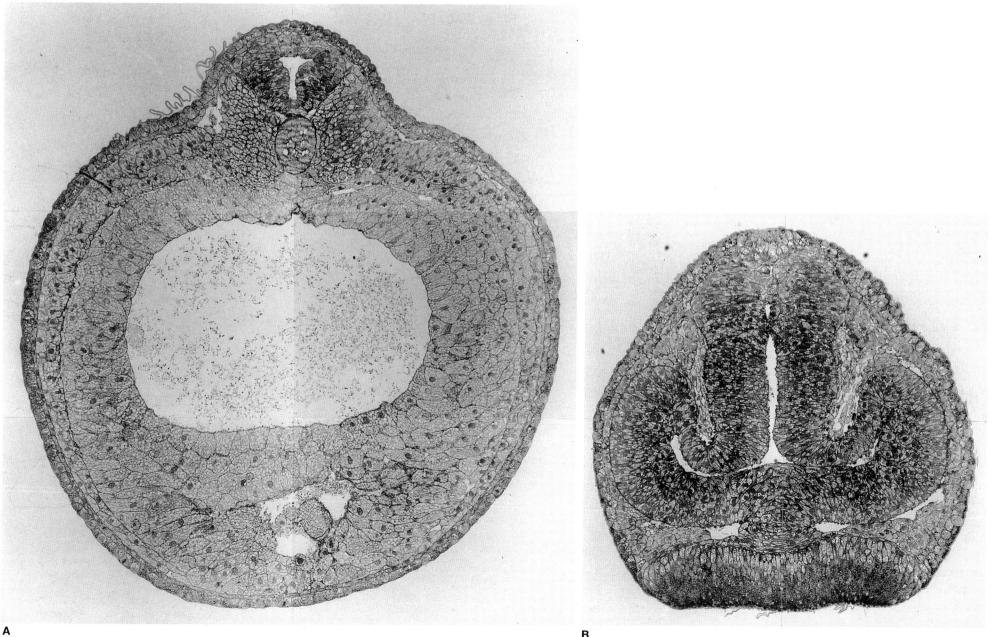

A

B

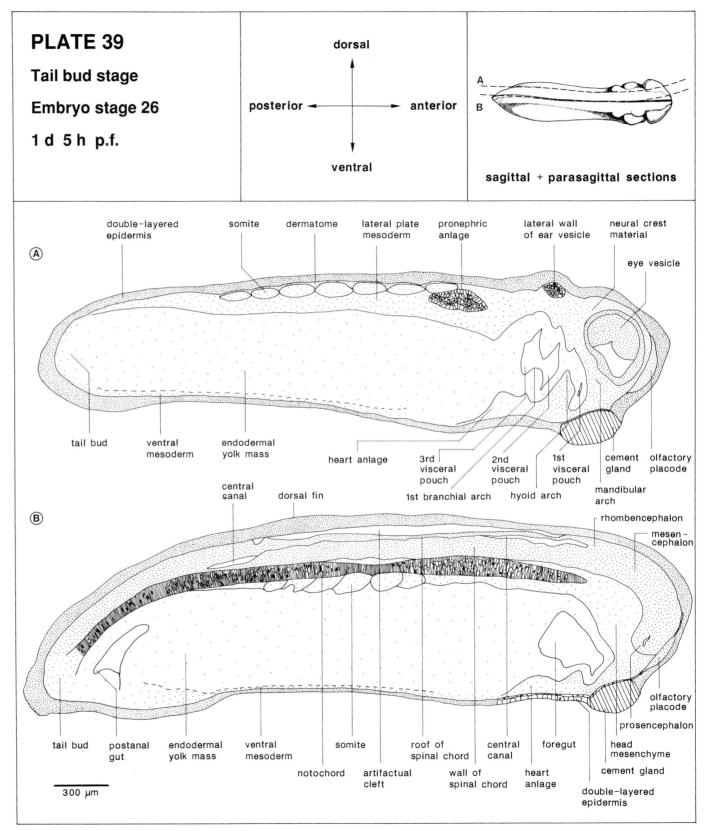

PLATE 39

Tail bud stage

Embryo stage 26

1 d 5 h p.f.

dorsal

posterior ← → anterior

ventral

sagittal + parasagittal sections

The Tail Bud Stage Embryo

The two sections were obtained from the same specimen. Due to a slight bending of the embryo the sections pass through the head region more laterally than through the trunk. A sagittal section through the head of the same specimen is given in PLATE 40B. (Staining: BCB)

(A)

double-layered epidermis — somite — dermatome — lateral plate mesoderm — pronephric anlage — lateral wall of ear vesicle — neural crest material — eye vesicle

tail bud — ventral mesoderm — endodermal yolk mass — heart anlage — 3rd visceral pouch — 2nd visceral pouch — 1st visceral pouch — cement gland — olfactory placode

1st branchial arch — hyoid arch — mandibular arch

(B)

central canal — dorsal fin — rhombencephalon — mesencephalon

tail bud — postanal gut — endodermal yolk mass — ventral mesoderm — somite — roof of spinal chord — central canal — foregut — olfactory placode

notochord — artifactual cleft — wall of spinal chord — heart anlage — prosencephalon — head mesenchyme — cement gland — double-layered epidermis

300 μm

PLATE 39

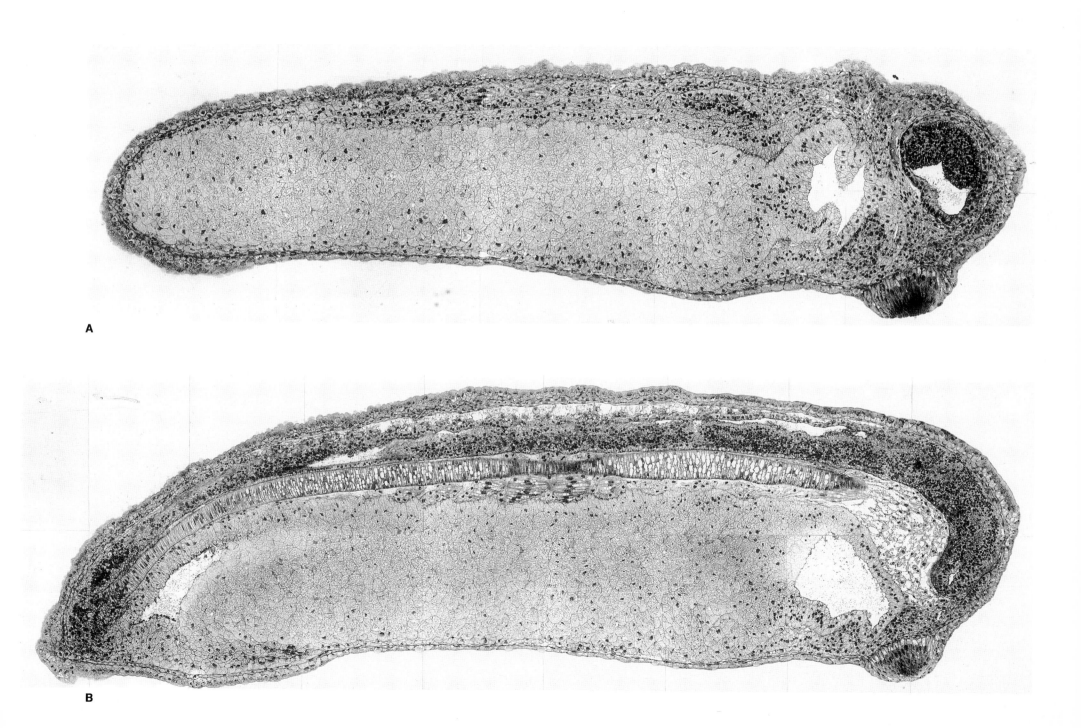

A

B

PLATE 40

Tail bud stage

Embryo stage 26

1 d 5 h p.f.

posterior ←——→ anterior

A

B

horizontal and sagittal sections

A Horizontal Section through the Head

The section passes through the brain and foregut of the embryo at a level just below the tip of the notochord and slightly above the ventral floor of the brain. The two massive eye anlagen evaginate from the diencephalon, the diencephalic ventricle extending into the eye vesicles. The connection between the brain and the eye vesicle represents the prospective optic stalk. The distal wall of the eye vesicle is in close contact with the epidermis. At this site the lens placode will form at stage 27 (cf. PLATE 42B). In front of the brain, between eye anlagen and the diencephalon, the sensorial layer of the epidermis has thickened to form the olfactory placodes. Posteriorly, the space between the brain and the adjacent archenteron wall is filled with head mesenchyme. (Staining: BCB)

B Sagittal Section through the Head

The cephalic flexure has reached an angle of about 90°. The brain ventricle has further enlarged. The dorsal roof and the ventral floor of the prosencephalon begin to thin out. The thickening of the anterior wall of the prosencephalon may represent the anlage of the olfactory lobe. The oral evagination approaches the ectoderm at the site of the future mouth opening. The columnar cells of the cement gland are clearly seen to be derived from the epithelial layer of the ectoderm. The notochord has become highly vacuolated. The heart anlage is clearly delimited in the ventral mesoderm. (Staining: BCB)

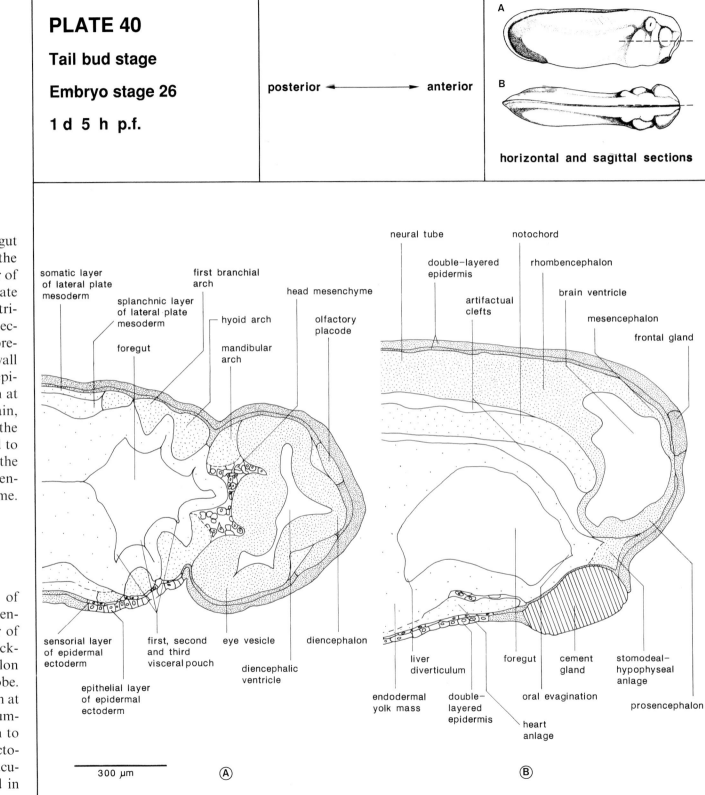

somatic layer of lateral plate mesoderm

splanchnic layer of lateral plate mesoderm

foregut

first branchial arch

hyoid arch

mandibular arch

head mesenchyme

olfactory placode

sensorial layer of epidermal ectoderm

epithelial layer of epidermal ectoderm

first, second and third visceral pouch

eye vesicle

diencephalic ventricle

diencephalon

neural tube

double-layered epidermis

artifactual clefts

notochord

rhombencephalon

brain ventricle

mesencephalon

frontal gland

endodermal yolk mass

double-layered epidermis

heart anlage

liver diverticulum

foregut

oral evagination

cement gland

stomodeal-hypophyseal anlage

prosencephalon

300 μm

Ⓐ

Ⓑ

PLATE 40

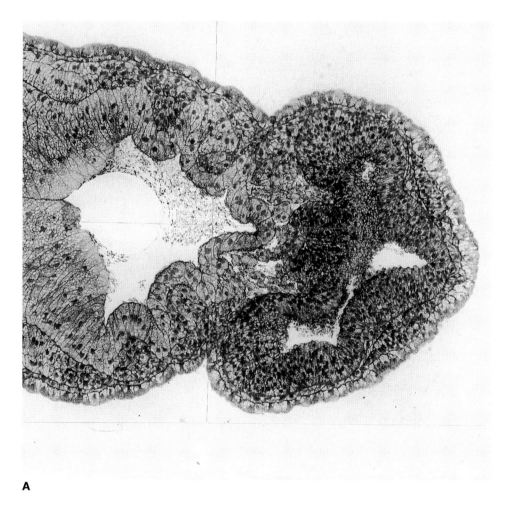

A

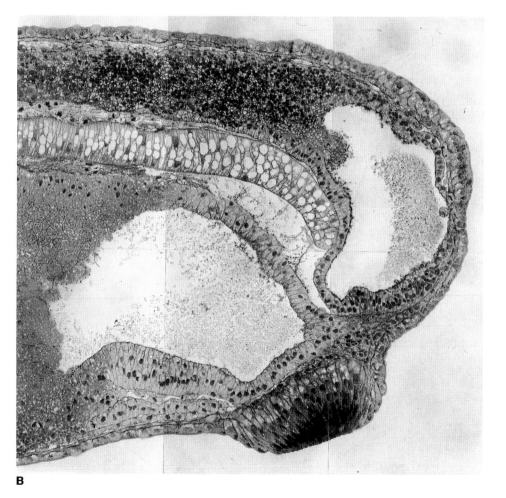

B

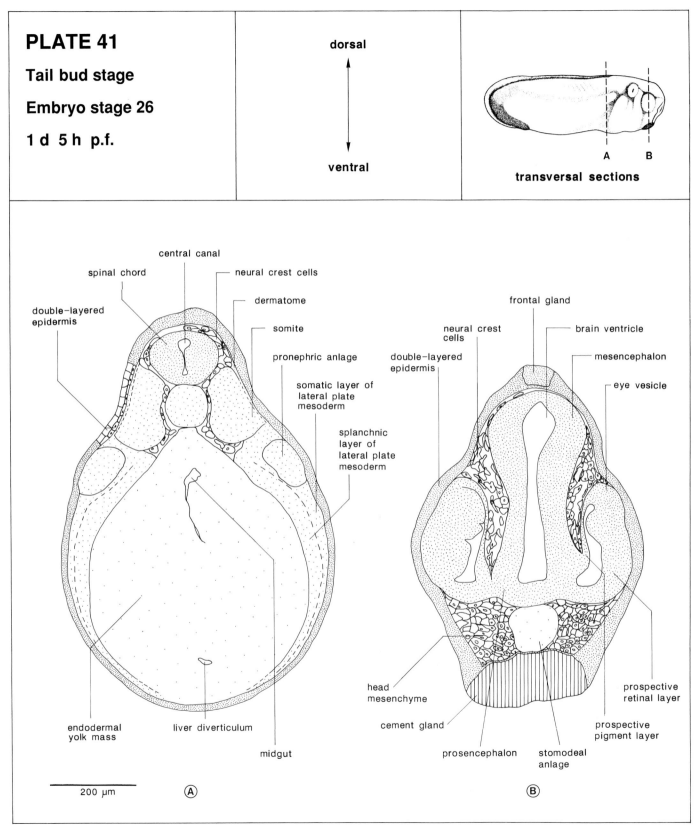

PLATE 41

Tail bud stage

Embryo stage 26

1 d 5 h p.f.

dorsal

ventral

transversal sections

central canal

spinal chord

neural crest cells

dermatome

double-layered epidermis

somite

pronephric anlage

somatic layer of lateral plate mesoderm

splanchnic layer of lateral plate mesoderm

frontal gland

neural crest cells

double-layered epidermis

brain ventricle

mesencephalon

eye vesicle

endodermal yolk mass

liver diverticulum

midgut

head mesenchyme

cement gland

prosencephalon

stomodeal anlage

prospective retinal layer

prospective pigment layer

200 μm

Ⓐ

Ⓑ

A Development of the Pronephros Continued

The pronephric anlage is fully segregated. It causes a slight bulge in the epidermis, which is visible externally. The neural tube and notochord become surrounded by cells which are probably of neural crest origin. The notochord has become highly vacuolated. The cavities in the endoderm represent the slit-shaped midgut and the liver diverticulum. (Staining: BCB)

B Development of the Eye Continued

The difference in thickness of the prospective retinal layer and the prospective pigment layer of the eye cup is more pronounced. The invagination of the eye vesicle begins. The eye anlagen are completely surrounded by neural crest material, which has filled all clefts and spaces in this region of the head. (Staining: BCB)

PLATE 41

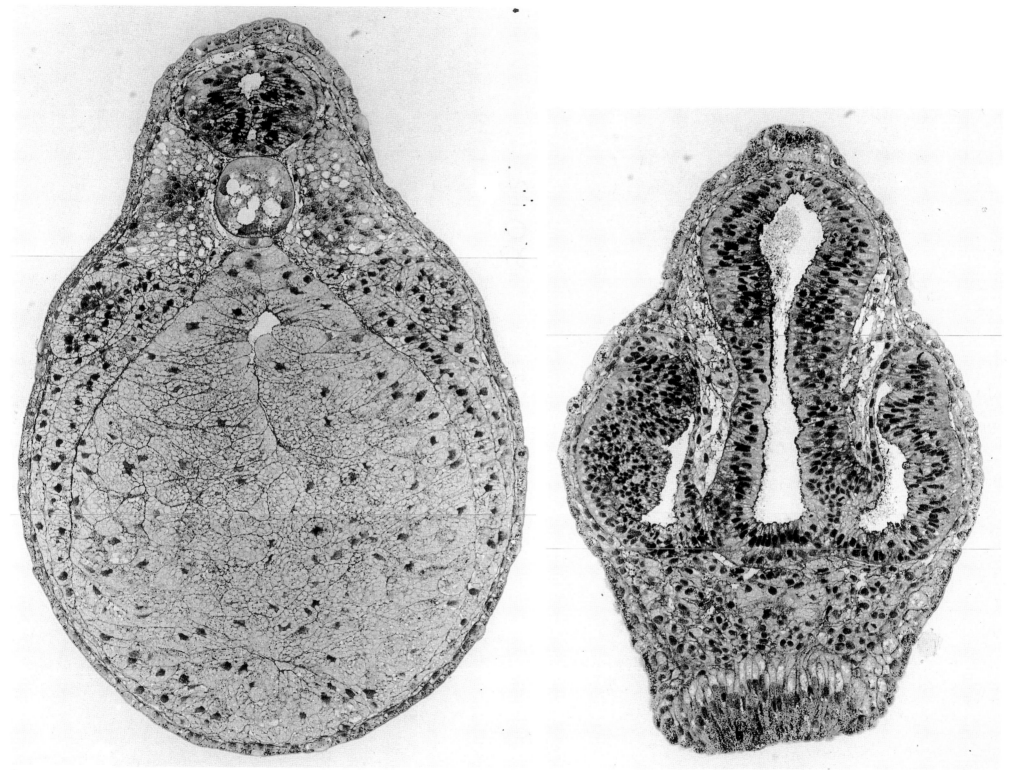

A

B

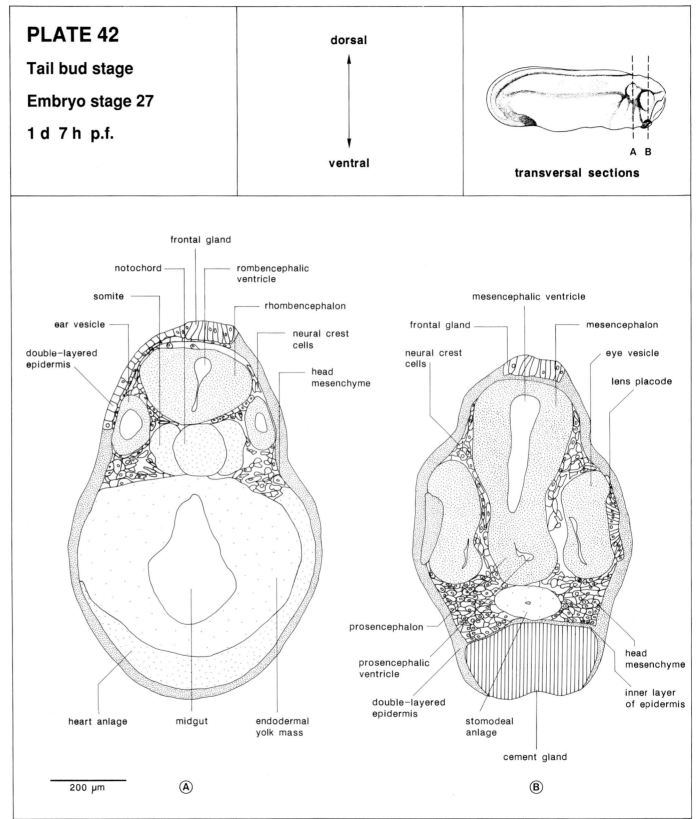

PLATE 42

Tail bud stage

Embryo stage 27

1 d 7 h p.f.

dorsal

ventral

A B

transversal sections

A The Ear Vesicle

The ear vesicle has formed from the sensorial layer of the epidermis in the rhombencephalic region of the head (cf. PLATE 43A-C). The notochord is surrounded by the most anterior part of the first pair of somites. On the *left side* the lateral endoderm of the first branchial pouch is in direct contact with the ectoderm to form the first branchial cleft. The heart anlage is indicated by the thickening of the ventrolateral mesoderm. (Staining: BCB)

B Lens Formation

Due to the cephalic flexure the section passes through the prosencephalon and the mesencephalon. The brain ventricle therefore appears as a long slit. The retinal layer of the eye vesicle begins to bend inwards to form the eye cup. Due to the beginning invagination of the eye vesicle, the retinal and pigment layers of the prospective retina approach each other, and the lumen of the eye vesicle is reduced. The lens placode has formed from the sensorial layer of the epidermis. (Staining: BCB)

frontal gland

notochord

rombencephalic ventricle

somite

rhombencephalon

ear vesicle

neural crest cells

double-layered epidermis

head mesenchyme

mesencephalic ventricle

frontal gland

mesencephalon

neural crest cells

eye vesicle

lens placode

prosencephalon

head mesenchyme

prosencephalic ventricle

double-layered epidermis

stomodeal anlage

inner layer of epidermis

cement gland

heart anlage

midgut

endodermal yolk mass

200 µm

Ⓐ

Ⓑ

PLATE 42

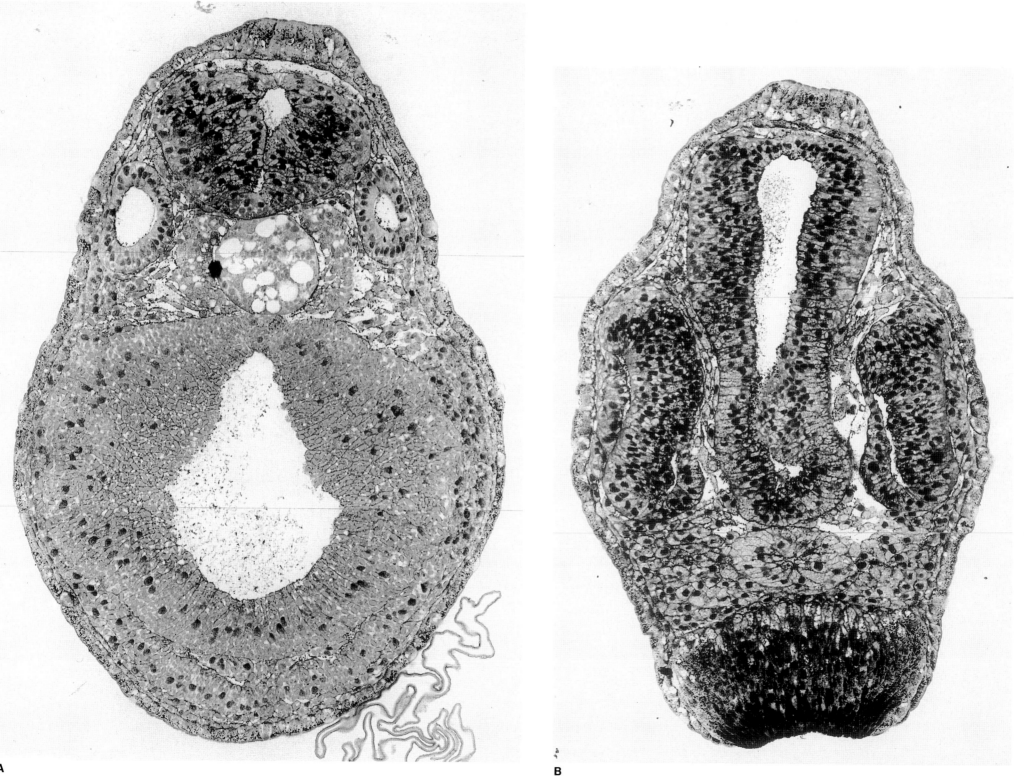

A

B

PLATE 43

Early Stages of Ear and Pronephros Development at Higher Magnification

A The Ear Anlage at Stage 21$^+$

The ear placode has formed in the sensorial layer of the epidermis. (Staining: BCB; magnification: 200x)

B The Ear Anlage at Stage 24

The invagination of the ear vesicle is underway. (Staining: BCB; magnification: 200x)

C The Ear Anlage at Stage 27

The ear vescicle is completely closed and has become detached from the sensorial layer of the epidermis. (Staining: BCB; magnification: 200x)

D The pronephric Anlage at Stage 21$^+$

The pronephric anlage is first visible as a thickening of the somatic layer of the lateral plate adjacent to the somite. (Staining: BCB; magnification: 200x)

E The Pronephric Anlage at Stage 24

A compact aggregate has formed. (Staining: BCB; magnification: 200x)

F The Pronephric Anlage at Stage 27

The cells within the aggregate have become arranged in a radial fashion. (Staining: BCB; magnification: 200x)

PLATE 43

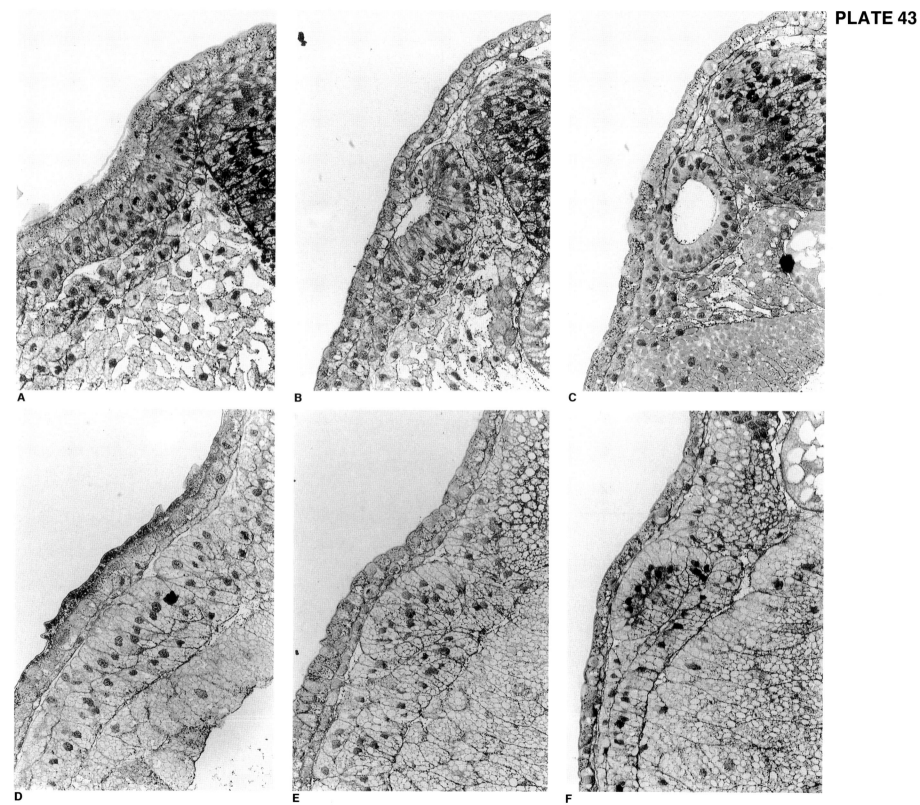

A

B

C

D

E

F

Index

This index lists the key terms used in the plates and allows crossreference to the text where they appear in bold face on the page indicated.

The copyright permission by the following companies to reproduce their figures is greatly acknowledged:

Academic Press, New York, U.S.A. (Figs. 3.3; 10.1; 10.2)
Cell Press, Cambridge MA, U.S.A. (Figs. 3.2; 6.1)
The Japanese Society of Developmental Biology, Tokyo, Japan (Fig. 3.4)
Elsevier Science Publishers, Amsterdam, Netherlands (graphics)
John Wiley & Sons Inc., New York, U.S.A. (Fig. 2.1)
The Company of Biologists Ltd., Cambridge, U.K. (Figs. 9.1; 9.3)
Springer Verlag GmbH, Heidelberg, F.R.G. (Fig. 5.2)
The Rockefeller University Press, New York, U.S.A. (Fig. 5.1)
Wissenschaftliche Verlagsgesellschaft, Stuttgart, F.R.G. (Fig. 3.1).